# Current Endovascular Treatment of Abdominal Aortic Aneurysms

# Current Endovascular Treatment of Abdominal Aortic Aneurysms

Edited by

## Albert G. Hakaim, MD

Consultant, Section of Vascular Surgery and Director,
Endovascular Surgery, Mayo Clinic, Jacksonville, Florida;
Associate Professor of Surgery, Mayo Clinic
College of Medicine, Rochester, Minnesota

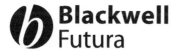

Nothing in this book implies endorsement by Mayo Foundation of products or companies mentioned.

The triple-shield Mayo logo and the words Mayo and Mayo Clinic are marks of Mayo Foundation for Medical Education and Research.

Published by Blackwell Publishing Ltd, 9600 Garsington Road, Oxford OX4 2DQ, UK
Printed and bound by Replika Press PVT. Ltd, India

Care has been taken to confirm the accuracy of the information presented and to describe generally accepted practices. However, the authors, editors, and publisher are not responsible for errors or omissions or for any consequences from application of the information in this book and make no warranty, express or implied, with respect to the contents of the publication. This book should not be relied on apart from the advice of a qualified health care provider.

The authors, editors, and publisher have exerted efforts to ensure that drug selection and dosage set forth in this text are in accordance with current recommendation and practice at the time of publication. However, in view of ongoing research, changes in government regulations, and the constant flow of information relating to drug therapy and drug reactions, the reader is urged to check the package insert for each drug for any change in indications and dosage and for added warnings and precautions. This is particularly important when the recommended agent is a new or infrequently employed drug.

Some drugs and medical devices presented in this publication have Food and Drug Administration (FDA) clearance for limited use in restricted research settings. It is the responsibility of the health care providers to ascertain the FDA status of each drug or device planned for use in their clinical practice.

Library of Congress Cataloging-in-Publication Data

Current endovascular treatment of abdominal aortic aneurysms / edited by Albert G. Hakaim.
  p. ; cm.
  Includes bibliographical references.
  ISBN-13: 978-1-4051-2205-4
  ISBN-10: 1-4051-2205-6
  1. Abdominal aneurysm–Endoscopic surgery.
  [DNLM: 1. Aortic Aneurysm, Abdominal–surgery. 2. Aortic Rupture–surgery. 3. Surgical Procedures, Operative–methods. WG 410 C976 2005] I. Hakaim, Albert G.

RD540.3.C87 2005
616.1'3307545–dc22

                                                                                    2005010453

A catalogue record for this title is available from the British Library

# Contents

# Contributors

**Perry S. Bechtle** DO
Consultant, Department of Anesthesiology,
Mayo Clinic, Jacksonville, Florida; Instructor in
Anesthesiology, Mayo Clinic College of Medicine,
Rochester, Minnesota

**Michael T. Caps** MD MPH
Division of Vascular Therapy, Hawaii
Permanente Medical Group, Honolulu, Hawaii

**Alfio Carroccio** MD
Assistant Professor, Department of Surgery,
Mount Sinai School of Medicine, New York, New
York

**Eric T. Choi** MD
Assistant Professor of Surgery and Radiology,
Washington University School of Medicine, St
Louis, Missouri

**Timothy A. M. Chuter** MD
Division of Vascular Surgery, University of
California, San Francisco, California

**Edward B. Diethrich** MD
Medical Director, Arizona Heart Institute and
Arizona Heart Hospital, Phoenix, Arizona

**Peter L. Faries** MD
Associate Professor, Department of Surgery, Weill
Medical College, New York, New York

**Richard J. Fowl** MD
Consultant, Division of General Surgery, Mayo
Clinic, Scottsdale, Arizona; Professor of Surgery,
Mayo Clinic College of Medicine, Rochester,
Minnesota

**Roy K. Greenberg** MD
Department of Vascular Surgery, Cleveland Clinic
Foundation, Cleveland, Ohio

**Albert G. Hakaim** MD
Consultant, Section of Vascular Surgery and
Director, Endovascular Surgery, Mayo Clinic,
Jacksonville, Florida; Associate Professor of
Surgery, Mayo Clinic College of Medicine,
Rochester, Minnesota

**William E. Haley** MD
Chair, Division of Nephrology and Hypertension,
Mayo Clinic, Jacksonville, Florida; Assistant
Professor of Medicine, Mayo Clinic College of
Medicine, Rochester, Minnesota

**Timothy A. Hipp** MD
Resident in Surgery, Mayo School of Graduate
Medical Education, Mayo Clinic College of
Medicine, Rochester, Minnesota

**Larry H. Hollier** MD
Professor and Chairman, Department of Surgery,
Mount Sinai School of Medicine, New York, New
York

**Eric A. Huettl** MD
Consultant, Department of Diagnostic Radiology,
Mayo Clinic, Scottsdale, Arizona; Assistant
Professor of Radiology, Mayo Clinic College of
Medicine, Rochester, Minnesota

**Krassi Ivancev** MD PhD
Endovascular Centre, Department of Radiology,
Malmö University Hospital, Malmö, Sweden

**Lisa Jordan** MSE
Spray Venture Partners, Newton, Massachusetts

**K. Craig Kent** MD
Professor of Surgery, Weill Cornell Medical
College; Chief, Division of Vascular Surgery, New
York Weill Cornell Medical Center & Columbia
Presbyterian Medical Center, New York, New
York

**Sashi Kilaru** MD
Vascular Surgery Fellow, New York Presbyterian
Hospital: Cornell Campus, New York, New York

**Josef Klocker** MD
Research Fellow in Vascular Research, Mayo
School of Graduate Medical Education, Mayo
Clinic College of Medicine, Rochester, Minnesota

## George E. Kopchok BS
Director, Vascular Surgery Research Laboratory, Division of Vascular Surgery, Harbor-UCLA Medical Center, Torrance, California

## L. Louis Lau MD FRCS
Vascular Research Fellow, Section of Vascular Surgery, Mayo Clinic, Jacksonville, Florida

## James T. Lee MD
Fellow, Vascular Surgery, Division of Vascular Surgery, Harbor-UCLA Medical Center, Torrance, California

## Bruce J. Leone MD
Consultant, Department of Anesthesiology, Mayo Clinic, Jacksonville, Florida; Associate Professor of Anesthesiology, Mayo Clinic College of Medicine, Rochester, Minnesota

## Martin Malina MD PhD
Endovascular Centre, Department of Radiology, Malmö University Hospital, Malmö, Sweden

## Michael L. Marin MD
Professor, Department of Surgery, Mount Sinai School of Medicine, New York, New York

## J. Mark McKinney MD
Consultant, Department of Radiology, Mayo Clinic, Jacksonville, Florida; Assistant Professor of Radiology, Mayo Clinic College of Medicine, Rochester, Minnesota

## Samuel R. Money MD FACS MBA
Head, Section of Vascular Surgery, Ochsner Clinic Foundation, Department of Surgery, New Orleans, Louisiana

## Monica Myers Mordecai MD
Senior Associate Consultant, Department of Anesthesiology, Mayo Clinic, Jacksonville, Florida; Instructor in Anesthesiology, Mayo Clinic College of Medicine, Rochester, Minnesota

## Thomas C. Naslund MD
Associate Professor of Surgery; Chief, Division of Vascular Surgery; Vanderbilt University School of Medicine, Nashville, Tennessee

## Beate Neuhauser MD
Vascular Research Fellow, Section of Vascular Surgery, Mayo Clinic, Jacksonville, Florida

## Audra A. Noel MD
Consultant, Division of Vascular Surgery, Mayo Clinic; Assistant Professor of Surgery, Mayo Clinic College of Medicine, Rochester, Minnesota

## Takao Ohki MD
Division of Vascular Surgery, Montefiore Medical Center and Albert Einstein College of Medicine, New York, New York

## W. Andrew Oldenburg MD
Head, Section of Vascular Surgery, Mayo Clinic, Jacksonville, Florida; Associate Professor of Surgery, Mayo Clinic College of Medicine, Rochester, Minnesota

## Ricardo Paz-Fumagalli MD
Consultant, Department of Radiology, Mayo Clinic, Jacksonville, Florida; Assistant Professor of Radiology, Mayo Clinic College of Medicine, Rochester, Minnesota

## Timothy M. Schmitt MD
Resident in Surgery, Mayo School of Graduate Medical Education, Mayo Clinic College of Medicine, Rochester, Minnesota

## Peter A. Schneider MD
Division of Vascular Therapy, Hawaii Permanente Medical Group, Honolulu, Hawaii

## Sherry D. Scovell MD
Vascular Surgery, Beth Israel Deaconess Medical Center, Boston, Massachusetts

## Gregario A. Sicard MD
Professor of Surgery and Radiology, Washington University School of Medicine, St Louis, Missouri

## Björn Sonesson MD PhD
Endovascular Centre, Department of Radiology, Malmö University Hospital, Malmö, Sweden

## Andrew H. Stockland MD
Senior Associate Consultant, Department of Radiology, Mayo Clinic, Jacksonville, Florida; Instructor in Radiology, Mayo Clinic College of Medicine, Rochester, Minnesota

## William M. Stone MD
Consultant, Division of General Surgery, Mayo Clinic, Scottsdale, Arizona; Associate Professor of Surgery, Mayo Clinic College of Medicine, Rochester, Minnesota

**Srinivasa Rao Vallabhaneni**
MD FRCS
Endovascular Centre, Department of Radiology,
Malmö University Hospital, Malmö, Sweden

**Frank J. Veith** MD
Division of Vascular Surgery, Montefiore Medical
Center and Albert Einstein College of Medicine,
New York, New York

**Andrew Wasiluk** MD
Consultant, Division of Nephrology and
Hypertension, Mayo Clinic, Jacksonville, Florida;
Assistant Professor of Medicine, Mayo Clinic
College of Medicine, Rochester, Minnesota

**Rodney A. White** MD
Professor of Surgery, UCLA School of Medicine;
Associate Chairman, Department of Surgery and
Chief, Division of Vascular Surgery, Harbor-
UCLA Medical Center; Torrance, California

**Jonathan D. Woody** MD
Assistant Professor of Surgery, Division of
Vascular Surgery, University of Pittsburgh School
of Medicine, University of Pittsburgh Medical
Center, Pittsburgh, Pennsylvania

**Osvaldo Juniti Yano** MD
Attending, St Francis Hospital, San Francisco,
California

**John W. York** MD
Department of Surgery, Section of Vascular
Surgery, Ochsner Clinic Foundation, New
Orleans, Louisiana

# Acknowledgments

My career in vascular surgery began at the Cleveland Clinic Foundation during the first day of my internship. From that time forward, my mentors have been Drs Norman R. Hertzer and Edwin G. Beven. Their skills and results were exemplary and remain the standard for traditional vascular surgical care.

Dr Alan Callow was instrumental in my visiting the University of Lund, at Malmö, Sweden, for an endovascular surgery fellowship with Dr Krassi Ivancev. His skills and results mirrored those of my earlier mentors and formed the basis for my continued interest in endovascular surgery.

Of course, my career and any accomplishments would not have been possible without the continued support and trust of Mayo Clinic and our patients.

Lastly, I thank my family for their support throughout my medical career.

A.G.H.

# Introduction

The incidence of vascular disease is expected to increase as life expectancy and the number of elderly people increase. For an aging patient population, endovascular techniques are appealing because they are minimally invasive. Many investigators have predicted that more than 80% of all vascular interventions will be replaced by endovascular techniques. Various catheter-based techniques have already been developed to treat the majority of vascular diseases, and major invasive operations have been replaced by procedures that use small incisions in remote arteries, which are used as access sites to deliver sophisticated devices to targets. In our endovascular center, my colleagues and I use endoluminal interventions daily to treat the majority of patients who have occlusive venous and arterial diseases, aneurysms, and vascular malformations.

The timing of a revolution could not be more appropriate. The feasibility trials for many of these endovascular interventions have already been successfully completed. Currently the Achilles heel of this technology is the durability of the repairs. However, one must realize that the technology is still in its embryonic phase and further understanding and developments are to come. Thus, continued rapid progress will improve clinical outcomes.

Undoubtedly, the delivery of care by the vascular specialist is also undergoing profound changes. Vascular surgeons and radiologists must merge their skills, perhaps developing a new discipline. This is an evolving process in which much of the training has to be done in a dichotomous fashion, with each type of specialist teaching the other.

Most importantly, we are living in a period of exciting transformation. The message for anyone interested in the treatment of vascular disease is to embrace the new endovascular techniques—learn them and improve them. This is the beginning of a new era.

A.G.H.

# PART I

## Preoperative and operative considerations

CHAPTER 1

# Long-term outcome following open repair of abdominal aortic aneurysms

**Audra A. Noel, MD**

## Introduction

Although endovascular repair has evolved as an important treatment method for patients with abdominal aortic aneurysm (AAA), open repair remains the standard. Comorbid factors, primarily coronary artery disease, affect the late outcome of AAA repair. Therefore, long-term results of endovascular repair should be compared with those of open repair. This chapter reviews the results of open repair of AAAs and the factors that affect morbidity and mortality.

## Operative mortality and morbidity

Elective repair of AAAs is accomplished by replacement of the aorta with a straight or bifurcated graft through a transperitoneal or retroperitoneal approach. In the past 20 years, large referral centers have reported mortality rates of 3–6%, despite the high incidence of preoperative comorbidities [1–4]. At Mayo Clinic, early mortality was 2.9% among 2452 patients undergoing elective repair of AAA between 1980 and 1990 [1]. The main causes of death among the 72 patients were cardiac (56%), respiratory (13%), and hemorrhagic (13%) conditions; gastrointestinal tract complications (11%); and stroke or sepsis (4%). When a subset of 400 consecutive elective cases (1980–85) was analyzed in a separate report, the mortality rate was 5.7% among high-risk patients and 1.7% among low-risk patients [5]. Hollier [6] reported on 100 high-risk patients who had one or more of the following characteristics: age older than 85 years, severe pulmonary disease, chronic renal failure, severe liver dysfunction, and severe cardiac disease. The mortality rate was 5%, and four of the five patients died of cardiac causes.

Other centers have achieved similar results. Cappeller *et al.* [3] reported an in-hospital mortality rate of 6.4% and a 30-day mortality rate of 4.9% for 545 consecutive patients treated for infrarenal aortic aneurysms between 1978 and 1987. Aune [4] reported that the 30-day mortality rate after AAA repair was 1.7% for a group of 118 patients younger than 66 years and 6% for patients 66 years or older.

Among patients undergoing repair of symptomatic, nonruptured AAAs, mortality is high (11.1%) [7]. Death at 60 days in this group was associated with emergency repair (performed within a few hours after admission), whereas no deaths were observed after semi-elective operations. When compared with the rate for elective repair, the major morbidity rate among patients with symptomatic, nonruptured AAA was significantly higher (47% vs 28%; $P < 0.05$) [7].

Moore *et al.* [8] compared 100 patients who had elective open AAA repair from 1992 to 1998 with a similar group of 100 patients who had elective endovascular repair. Although the surgical mortality rate was not significantly less in the endovascular group than in the open repair group (2% vs 3%), the benefits of endovascular repair included less surgical time, less blood loss and replacement, less need for intensive care, and shorter duration of total hospital stay. Patients with endovascular repair tended to have lower morbidity rates for myocardial infarction (1% vs 5%), respiratory failure (1% vs 5%), and colon ischemia (0% vs 2%).

## Factors affecting long-term survival

Late survival is predominantly determined by cardiac status. Overall 5-year survival ranges from 61% to 79% and is significantly less than for age- and sex-matched controls in most studies (Table 1.1) [2,3,9–12]. When compared directly, 5-year survival after endovascular repair (65%) and 5-year survival after open repair (72%) are equivalent [8].

Hollier *et al.* [2] reported long-term follow-up of 1087 patients who underwent either elective or ruptured AAA repair: survival rates were 68% at 5 years and 41% at 10 years (Table 1.1). The cause of death was cardiac-related for 38% of the patients, whereas neoplasm caused 15% of the deaths, ruptured aneurysm 8%, and stroke 7%. Advanced age and heart disease or hyperten-

**Table 1.1** Long-term survival after open repair of abdominal aortic aneurysms.

| Authors; year of publication | 5-year survival, % | 10-year survival, % | Predictors of late death |
|---|---|---|---|
| Hollier *et al.*; 1984 [2] | 67.5 | 40.7 | Age, hypertension, CAD* |
| Koskas & Kieffer; 1997 [9] | 66.9 | – | Multiple, including age, CAD, renal failure |
| Norman *et al.*; 1998 [10] | 79 | – | |
| Cappeller *et al.*; 1998 [3] | 65 | 41 | Age, hypertension, CAD |
| Yasuhara *et al.*; 1999 [11] | 61–73 | – | Renal dysfunction, pulmonary dysfunction |
| Komori *et al.*; 1999 [12] | 71 | 52 | Age, renal dysfunction, pulmonary dysfunction |

*CAD, coronary artery disease.

sion significantly correlated with shorter survival time. Of the patients who survived AAA repair, 12% subsequently died of rupture of another aneurysm or of late complication of the aneurysm repair, suggesting the need for long-term monitoring. For patients without preoperative hypertension or heart disease, duration of survival was comparable to that of an age- and sex-matched general population group.

Koskas & Kieffer [9] compiled data from all open, elective aneurysms repaired in 28 centers in 1989 (834 procedures). Again, the mean annual death rate from cardiovascular death was higher for AAA repair patients (1.8%) than for the control group. In addition, multiple anatomical and perioperative factors such as diameter of aneurysm, choice of surgical approach, left ventricular insufficiency, carotid occlusion, cardiac arrhythmia, myocardial infarction on electrocardiography, abnormal aorta cephalad to the aneurysm, and renal insufficiency were independent predictors of late death (Table 1.1). These data suggest that control of perioperative factors and long-term monitoring for cardiac dysfunction are important for late survival.

Because of the high incidence of late cardiac-related deaths among patients with open AAA repair, the question of preoperative cardiac revascularization has been entertained. To evaluate the effect on late survival of using selective myocardial revascularization with coronary artery bypass grafting, records were reviewed from 485 patients who had AAA repair from 1980 to 1985 at Mayo Clinic [13]. The late survival of the treated groups with uncorrected or bypassed cardiac disease was not significantly different from that of a matched population, whereas patients without coronary artery disease had a higher 5-year survival rate than the general population (83% vs 76%). This study is one of the few that show improved survival rates for patients who had AAA repair as compared with controls, possibly because of the use of selective preoperative myocardial revascularization with bypass [13]. Although preoperative percutaneous transluminal coronary angioplasty may confer protection against cardiac events in the perioperative period, this procedure is associated with a higher incidence of late cardiac events than coronary bypass, possibly because of stent restenosis [1].

Yasuhara et al. [11] reported results from 338 consecutive patients treated with elective repair between 1980 and 1997. In this series, a history of cardiac disease predicted only cardiac-related death. Renal dysfunction and a history of cerebrovascular events, however, were predictive of decreased long-term survival. Komori et al. [12] found that renal dysfunction, in addition to pulmonary dysfunction and age, was a significant negative predictor of long-term survival for a group of 332 patients who had elective, open AAA repair. Treatment of patients with renal failure or insufficiency is particularly challenging because of concomitant renovascular hypertension, the potential need for suprarenal aortic clamp placement, and perioperative fluid management. Endovascular repair with the use of nephrotoxic contrast medium may not be an appropriate option for patients with renal insufficiency. Instead, other means of non-nephrotoxic aortic imaging, such as intravascular ultrasonography or gadolinium-based imaging, may be useful.

Age and sex also influence late survival. Aune [4] found that the postoperative 8-year survival of patients younger than 66 years was 69%, which was significantly less than that for a demographically matched population. By comparison, 8-year survival for patients 66 years or older was 47%, which, although lower, is a better relative survival than that for the younger group ($P < 0.05$). Reigel et al. [13] also noted significantly worse late survival for patients in their 50s and 60s than for a matched population. However, octogenarians undergoing elective AAA repair had the same late survival as a matched population [10,13]. Therefore, age alone should not be a contraindication for open AAA repair. Norman et al. [10] noted that relative 5-year survival after AAA repair was 88% for women and 95% for men. After repair of ruptured AAA, women had higher mortality than men [14,15]. The reason for a difference between sexes is unclear but may be related to a higher incidence of cardiovascular disease in women than expected. In future studies, sex should be considered when comparing open repair with endovascular repair.

In the series of 545 patients studied by Cappeller et al. [3], late mortality most frequently resulted from cardiac disease (49%) and malignancy (13%). Only 5 of the 545 patients died of vascular-related complications such as new or recurrent aneurysm. Other series have also had a high incidence (13–30%) of malignancy-related deaths after open AAA repair, suggesting that concomitant cancer-screening should be included in the follow-up of this patient population [2,9,10,16,17].

## Graft-related complications and recurrent aneurysms

The necessity for long-term surveillance of graft-related complications is an important consideration when comparing open AAA repair with endovascular repair. Hallett et al. [18] reported on 307 patients in one community who were followed up between 1957 and 1990 (mean duration of follow-up, 5.8 years). The most common complications were anastomotic pseudoaneurysm (3%, at a median follow-up of 6.1 years), graft thrombosis (2%; median, 0.9 year), graft–enteric erosion or fistula (1.7%; median, 4.3 years), graft infection (1.6%; median, 0.2 year), anastomotic hemorrhage (1.3%; median, 0.1 year), and colon ischemia (0.7%) and atheroembolism (0.3%) in the first 30 days postoperatively [18]. Because anastomotic pseudoaneurysm was the most common complication, the authors recommended graft surveillance with ultrasonography or computed tomography at 1 year and then every 3–5 years. The low incidence of graft-related complications is reassuring.

The presence of late anastomotic aneurysms with changes in aortic or iliac size raises concerns about the security of the endograft attachment many years after the operation. In a population-based analysis of 432 patients (mean duration of follow-up, 6 years), new aortic aneurysms occurred in the proximal aorta in 5% of the patients who had tube graft repairs and in 2.5% of the patients who had bifurcated graft repairs [19]. No clinically evident or autopsy-proven iliac aneurysms or iliac occlusive disease occurred, however, in the patients treated with tube grafts. These data suggest that open treatment of AAAs with straight grafts when feasible offers limited dissection without concern for late iliac disease. Sonesson *et al.* [20] evaluated the progression of aortic neck size among 19 patients undergoing open repair from 1989 to 1993; they found that the infrarenal aorta enlarged at a rate of 0.5 mm annually after repair. The data suggested that two groups may exist—one with a low aortic growth rate and one with a higher rate. Unfortunately, no distinguishing characteristics could be identified to select these patients preoperatively. If selection criteria could be determined, patients with a higher rate of annual aortic growth may be identified as being less suitable for endograft repair.

## Quality of life

The quality of life for patients undergoing AAA repair has not been well documented, although with the advent of less invasive repair, quality of life is a crucial point of comparison. The United Kingdom Small Aneurysm Trial Participants used the Medical Outcomes Study questionnaire to score health-related quality of life for 1090 patients preoperatively and up to 1 year postoperatively [21]. Patients undergoing early open repair, as compared with observation, had significant improvement in health perceptions and bodily pain. Although these differences were small, the data raise more questions about the evaluation of quality of life for patients undergoing AAA repair. Future comparisons of open and endovascular AAA repair should include such data.

## Ruptured aneurysms

Ruptured aneurysms remain lethal despite advances in hospital transportation and critical care management. Overall mortality ranges from 45% to 70% for patients who present to the hospital, with little improvement over the past 2 decades [14,22–25]. In the Mayo Clinic series of 413 patients managed for ruptured AAAs during an 18-year period, women and patients older than 80 years had a higher mortality rate [14]. Therefore, women and elderly patients with ruptured AAAs may benefit from endovascular repair in the future.

Late complications in 116 patients treated for ruptured AAAs were evaluated by Cho *et al.* [26]. Median duration of follow-up was >7 years. At 1, 5, and 10 years, survival rates were 86%, 64%, and 33%, respectively, which were significantly lower than for patients treated with elective AAA repair (97%, 74%, and 43%; $P = 0.02$) and for the general population (95%, 75%, and 52%; $P < 0.001$). Patients with ruptured AAAs had a higher incidence of paraanastomotic aneurysms, but coronary artery disease was the most frequent cause of death in both the ruptured AAA and the elective repair groups.

Because patients who have a ruptured AAA have a higher incidence of vascular and graft-related complications (20 of 116; 17%) than patients who have elective AAA repair (9 of 116; 8%), patients surviving ruptured AAA repair should be monitored closely. Of course, elective repair is preferred when possible, but because two-thirds of patients who survive ruptured AAA repair are alive 5 years after the operation, aggressive surgical intervention is indicated.

## Summary

Open repair of AAAs is the standard, with low morbidity and mortality and few long-term graft complications, despite relatively decreased survival owing to cardiac complications. Patients with severe cardiac dysfunction, women, and patients with symptomatic or ruptured AAAs have decreased survival after open repair and may benefit from preferential use of endovascular repair.

## References

1 Elmore JR, Hallett JW Jr, Gibbons RJ et al. Myocardial revascularization before abdominal aortic aneurysmorrhaphy: effect of coronary angioplasty. Mayo Clin Proc 1993; **68**: 637–41.

2 Hollier LH, Plate G, O'Brien PC et al. Late survival after abdominal aortic aneurysm repair: influence of coronary artery disease. J Vasc Surg 1984; **1**: 290–9.

3 Cappeller WA, Holzel D, Hinz MH, Lauterjung L. Ten-year results following elective surgery for abdominal aortic aneurysm. Int Angiol 1998; **17**: 234–40.

4 Aune S. Risk factors and operative results of patients aged less than 66 years operated on for asymptomatic abdominal and aortic aneurysm. Eur J Vasc Endovasc Surg 2001; **22**: 240–3.

5 Hollier LH, Reigel MM, Kazmier FJ et al. Conventional repair of abdominal aortic aneurysm in the high-risk patient: a plea for abandonment of nonresective treatment. J Vasc Surg 1986; **3**: 712–17.

6 Hollier LH. Surgical management of abdominal aortic aneurysm in the high-risk patient. Surg Clin North Am 1986; **66**: 269–79.

7 Cambria RA, Gloviczki P, Stanson AW et al. Symptomatic, nonruptured abdominal aortic aneurysms: are emergent operations necessary? Ann Vasc Surg 1994; **8**: 121–6.

8 Moore WS, Kashyap VS, Vescera CL, Quinones-Baldrich WJ. Abdominal aortic aneurysm: a 6-year comparison of endovascular versus transabdominal repair. Ann Surg 1999; **230**: 298–306.

9 Koskas F, Kieffer E, for the Association for Academic Research in Vascular Surgery (AURC). Long-term survival after elective repair of infrarenal abdominal aortic aneurysm: results of a prospective multicentric study. Ann Vasc Surg 1997; **11**: 473–81.

10 Norman PE, Semmens JB, Lawrence-Brown MM, Holman CD. Long term relative survival after surgery for abdominal aortic aneurysm in western Australia: population based study. BMJ 1998; **317**: 852–6.

11 Yasuhara H, Ishiguro T, Muto T. Factors affecting late survival after elective abdominal aortic aneurysm repair. Br J Surg 1999; **86**: 1047–52.

12 Komori K, Takeuchi K, Ohta S *et al.* Factors influencing late survival after abdominal aortic aneurysm repair in Japanese patients. *Surgery* 1999; **125**: 545–52.

13 Reigel MM, Hollier LH, Kazmier FJ *et al.* Late survival in abdominal aortic aneurysm patients: the role of selective myocardial revascularization on the basis of clinical symptoms. *J Vasc Surg* 1987; **5**: 222–7.

14 Noel AA, Gloviczki P, Cherry KJ Jr *et al.* Ruptured abdominal aortic aneurysms: the excessive mortality rate of conventional repair. *J Vasc Surg* 2001; **34**: 41–6.

15 Semmens JB, Norman PE, Lawrence-Brown MM, Holman CD. Influence of gender on outcome from ruptured abdominal aortic aneurysm. *Br J Surg* 2000; **87**: 191–4.

16 Norman PE, Semmens JB, Lawrence-Brown MM. Long-term relative survival following surgery for abdominal aortic aneurysm: a review. *Cardiovasc Surg* 2001; **9**: 219–24.

17 Johnston KW, and the Canadian Society for Vascular Surgery Aneurysm Study Group. Nonruptured abdominal aortic aneurysm: six-year follow-up results from the multicenter prospective Canadian aneurysm study. *J Vasc Surg* 1994; **20**: 163–70.

18 Hallett JW Jr, Marshall DM, Petterson TM *et al.* Graft-related complications after abdominal aortic aneurysm repair: reassurance from a 36-year population-based experience. *J Vasc Surg* 1997; **25**: 277–84.

19 Calcagno D, Hallett JW Jr, Ballard DJ *et al.* Late iliac artery aneurysms and occlusive disease after aortic tube grafts for abdominal aortic aneurysm repair: a 35-year experience. *Ann Surg* 1991; **214**: 733–6.

20 Sonesson B, Resch T, Lanne T, Ivancev K. The fate of the infrarenal aortic neck after open aneurysm surgery. *J Vasc Surg* 1998; **28**: 889–94.

21 UK Small Aneurysm Trial Participants. Health service costs and quality of life for early elective surgery or ultrasonographic surveillance for small abdominal aortic aneurysms. *Lancet* 1998; **352**: 1656–60.

22 Gloviczki P, Pairolero P, Mucha P Jr *et al.* Ruptured abdominal aortic aneurysms: repair should not be denied. *J Vasc Surg* 1992; **15**: 851–7.

23 Johansen K, Kohler TR, Nicholls SC *et al.* Ruptured abdominal aortic aneurysm: the Harborview experience. *J Vasc Surg* 1991; **13**: 240–5.

24 McCready RA, Siderys H, Pittman JN *et al.* Ruptured abdominal aortic aneurysms in a private hospital: a decade's experience (1980–1989). *Ann Vasc Surg* 1993; **7**: 225–8.

25 Milner QJ, Burchett KR. Long-term survival following emergency abdominal aortic aneurysm repair. *Anaesthesia* 2000; **55**: 432–5.

26 Cho JS, Gloviczki P, Martelli E *et al.* Long-term survival and late complications after repair of ruptured abdominal aortic aneurysms. *J Vasc Surg* 1998; **27**: 813–19.

CHAPTER 2

# Durability of endovascular repair of infrarenal aortoiliac aneurysms: what lessons have been learned?

**Josef Klocker, MD, Albert G. Hakaim, MD**

## Introduction

New concepts and techniques that are introduced as alternatives to conventional treatment strategies may have advantageous effects (justifying their application) as well as new risks (limiting their application), which may be previously unknown and unexpected. Therefore, critical data analysis, rigorous review, and follow-up of patients are crucial to define or redefine indications for treatment using any technique.

Immediate technical and clinical success rates are promising for endovascular aneurysm repair (EVAR) of aortic aneurysms, particularly for the treatment of patients at high risk for open surgery. It was presumed that EVAR would be economical and that it would provide better survival than open repair of abdominal aortic aneurysm (AAA) [1]. Long-term durability and long-term success of EVAR (defined as outcome measures beyond 5 years [2]), however, are not definitively established because data on long-term follow-up of patients undergoing EVAR are not yet available.

## Outcome criteria: how to define success of AAA repair

In general, primary outcome criteria after aneurysm repair include (1) prevention of aneurysmal rupture; (2) prevention of death from rupture; (3) prevention of death from primary and secondary interventions [2]. Previous AAA treatment, using either open repair or EVAR, does not necessarily prohibit subsequent aneurysmal rupture or aneurysm-related death (owing to, for example, ruptured pseudoaneurysm or graft infection in patients who underwent open repair). Therefore, secondary outcome criteria include surrogate markers that suggest a continuing or increasing risk of rupture, such as endoleak, endotension, changes in the AAA diameter, and freedom from secondary interventions.

An endoleak is defined as the presence of blood flow outside the lumen of the endoluminal graft but within the aneurysm sac, as determined by an imaging study [2,3]. Endoleaks indicate incomplete exclusion of the aneurysm resulting from an incomplete seal between the endograft and the wall of the blood vessel (type I endoleak), retrograde blood flow from patent aortic side branches (type II), inadequate connection between components of a modular prosthesis or fabric disruption (type III), or device porosity (type IV).

Endotension is a state of increased pressure within the aneurysm sac [2,4]. Persistent or recurrent pressurization of the aneurysm could result either from blood flow that is not detectable with the sensitivity limits of current imaging technology or from pressure transmission through a thrombus or endograft fabric. At present, "endotension" is an investigative term and, because direct intrasac pressure measurement is not available for routine follow-up, there is disagreement about its precise definition, appropriate usage, and current applicability. According to the "Reporting Standards for Endovascular Aortic Aneurysm Repair" [2], the term "endotension" should be used only to describe instances of aneurysmal enlargement after EVAR in the absence of a detectable endoleak.

Changes in the dimension of the aortic aneurysm affect the outcome assessment. Aneurysmal growth after EVAR is an indicator of incomplete exclusion of the aneurysm, continued risk of aneurysmal rupture, and a presumed treatment failure [5].

To meet the primary goal of aneurysm repair (i.e., to prevent rupture), primary adjunctive procedures (i.e., at the time of the original operation), secondary adjunctive procedures (i.e., on a subsequent occasion), or conversion to open repair may be indicated in the absence of technically or clinically successful aneurysm repair. These procedures may be associated with additional morbidity and mortality and are therefore considered to be important parameters of outcome analysis.

## The EUROSTAR registry: multicenter outcome analysis of EVAR

In 1996, the EUROSTAR registry was established to provide data on early and late outcomes after EVAR. Before AAA repair, patients with AAA suitable for EVAR were included in a data registry center. Data were collected for the following: demographic characteristics, anatomical characteristics of the aneurysms, details of the device used, complications encountered during the procedure, immediate outcome, all adverse events, and results of contrast-enhanced computed tomographic imaging at 3, 6, 12, and 18 months and yearly thereafter.

Extensive reports on the outcome of EVAR taken from the EUROSTAR database were written by Harris et al. [6] and van Marrewijk et al. [7]. Harris and coworkers [6] analyzed records from a total of 2464 patients who had been included on an intention-to-treat basis in 88 centers in 16 European countries (male:female ratio, 11.5:1; mean age, 70.5 years; age range, 37–93 years). Among these patients, 652 (26.5%) had undergone previous laparotomy, but only 320 (13.0%) were considered to be unfit for conventional open surgery.

Even though the mean (± SD) duration of follow-up was only 12.2 ± 12.3 months, the follow-up period extended to 4 years for some individuals.

## Aneurysmal rupture after EVAR and rupture-related mortality

### Risk and outcome of late aneurysmal rupture after EVAR

Lumsden et al. [8] first reported that risk of rupture may persist after EVAR. Rupture risk was quantified by the EUROSTAR registry analysis [6]. In the series of 2464 patients, 13 (0.5%) had unequivocal evidence of rupture of a treated aneurysm 30 days or more after EVAR (Table 2.1). The peak incidence of rupture occurred 18 months after the operation; the cumulative risk of rupture was approximately 1% per year. As stated by Harris and coworkers [6], the calculated risk of rupture would increase to 1.7% per year if patients who died suddenly of unconfirmed causes, possibly owing to rupture, were included as well. It was assumed that these results reflected complications of treatment mainly using the earliest generation of endovascular devices, such as early models of endovascular aortic grafts that were withdrawn subsequently. It is possible that newer generations of endografts will perform differently, but this remains to be proved.

In the EUROSTAR series of 11 patients who underwent emergency open repair for late rupture after EVAR, five (45.4%) survived. Another two patients who were not operated on died. The overall mortality from late rupture was 61.5% (8 of 13), which is comparable to the death rates of open repair in ruptured and previously untreated AAAs [9].

### Risk factors for late aneurysmal rupture after EVAR

Significant risk factors for late rupture in the EUROSTAR experience published by Harris and coworkers [6] were proximal type I endoleak ($P = 0.001$),

**Table 2.1** Outcome after endovascular aneurysm repair of abdominal aortic aneurysms as calculated in the EUROSTAR registry of 2464 patients.

| End point | Patients | | Cumulative risk per year, % | Mortality, % |
|---|---|---|---|---|
| | No. | % | | |
| Late rupture*† | 13 | 0.5 | 1.0–1.7 | 61.5 |
| Endoleak | | | | |
| Overall‡ | 488 | 19.8 | – | – |
| At 1 month‡ | 171 | 6.9 | – | – |
| De novo‡ | 317 | 12.9 | – | – |
| Late conversion†§ | 41 | 1.7 | 2.1 | 24.4 |

*Rupture occurring 30 days or more after repair.
†Mean (± SD) duration of follow-up, 12.2 ± 12.3 months [6].
‡Mean duration of follow-up, 15.4 months (range, 1–72 months) [7].
§Conversion occurring more than 30 days after repair.

midgraft type III endoleak ($P = 0.001$), graft migration ($P = 0.001$), and post-operative kinking of the endograft ($P = 0.001$). There was no association of late ruptures with distal type I endoleak ($P = 0.776$), type II endoleak ($P = 0.415$), endograft stenosis ($P = 0.646$), or thrombosed endograft ($P = 0.503$).

The EUROSTAR experience with endoleaks during follow-up was summarized in detail by van Marrewijk *et al.* [7]. The overall prevalence of endoleaks was approximately 20% (Table 2.1), which is in agreement with persistent endoleak rates observed in other studies [5]. In 7% of the patients, endoleaks were present at the first-month postoperative visit, whereas in 13% they developed later during follow-up. Matsumura & Moore [5] observed a greater tendency for growth in aneurysms with *de novo* endoleaks, and these authors suggested that this category includes a separate type of endoleak.

The EUROSTAR analysis certainly highlights the major importance of proximal fixation-site endoleaks (type Ia). Secondary interventions, either endovascular or open, are mandatory to correct this problem. By contrast, distal fixation-site endoleaks (type Ib) seem to have no effect on the risk of rupture. Unfortunately, whereas most distal fixation-site endoleaks are repaired quite easily using minor secondary endovascular procedures, proximal fixation-site endoleaks are comparatively difficult to treat.

The EUROSTAR experience showed no significant correlation of type II endoleaks with late aneurysmal rupture. According to anecdotal evidence, however, type II endoleaks are responsible for late rupture after EVAR; therefore, the management of active side branches is still a matter of extensive discussion. Conflicting opinions range from a strictly conservative policy to active obliteration by coil embolization.

## Late conversion to open repair

Harris and coworkers [6] showed that the cumulative risk of late conversion is approximately 2.1% per year (Table 2.1). Interestingly, the risk increased with time after the operation: the risk was 1% in the first year and 3.7% in the second year. In general, the decision to remove and replace an endovascular device with a conventionally sutured graft does not follow standardized rules. It should be directed by the fact that the risk of rupture and rupture-related death can be estimated in cases of known technical or clinical failures of treatment. Risk factors in these cases may be regarded as indications for late conversion. As stated by Harris and coworkers [6], the risk of aneurysmal rupture or other life- or limb-threatening disaster must be substantially greater than the risk of conversion before this course of action should be recommended to the patient.

### Freedom from secondary intervention in patients with or without endoleaks

Life table analysis of the EUROSTAR data showed a freedom-from-secondary-intervention rate that was significantly less for patients with endoleak than for patients without endoleak ($P$ = 0.001). At 2 years, the rates were 61.1% for 191 patients (7.8% of the whole study cohort) with type II endoleak; 41.1% for 297 patients (12.0% of the cohort) with type I, type III, or multiple endoleaks; and 91.3% for 1975 patients (80.2% of the cohort) who never had an endoleak [7]. These data indicate that there is a substantial risk of secondary interventions only if endoleaks are present and that the rate of secondary procedures is significantly less for patients with type II endoleak than for patients with type I or type III endoleak. This may reflect different strategies and the ongoing discussion about the treatment of type II endoleaks.

Ohki and coworkers [10] reported on 25 secondary interventions in a series of 239 patients (mean ± SD duration of follow-up, 15.7 ± 6.3 months). The interventions were required for the following reasons: endoleak type I ($n$ = 7), type II ($n$ = 6), or type III ($n$ = 1); graft thrombosis ($n$ = 5); iliac artery stenosis ($n$ = 2); aortoenteric fistula ($n$ = 2); and aneurysmal rupture ($n$ = 2). Three patients (13%) died: both patients who underwent conversion for aortoenteric fistula repair and one patient after aneurysmal rupture.

### Outcome of late conversion to open repair

In the EUROSTAR experience, 41 patients underwent late conversion to open repair. The perioperative mortality rate was 24.4%, which is approximately six times higher than that associated with primary open repair of an abdominal aortic aneurysm. The peak incidence of conversion, at the time of analysis, occurred at 18 months (range, 1–48 months).

### Risk factors for late conversion to open repair

Significant risk factors for late conversion were proximal type I endoleak ($P$ = 0.001), midgraft type III endoleak ($P$ = 0.001), type II endoleak ($P$ = 0.003), graft migration ($P$ = 0.001), graft kinking ($P$ = 0.001), and distal type I endoleak ($P$ = 0.001). Nonsignificant indications for late conversion were endograft stenosis ($P$ = 0.662) and thrombosed endografts ($P$ = 0.148) [6].

A proximal fixation-site endoleak that cannot be resolved by other means is universally acknowledged to be a compelling indication for conversion. Its strong association with rupture confirms the appropriateness of this approach. Stent migration may necessitate conversion because this is an important cause of proximal fixation-site endoleaks. However, it is not universally accepted that endoleaks from other sites inevitably warrant conversion. For type II endoleaks, conversion is not justified unless there is also evidence of continuing expansion of the aneurysm sac. Similarly, endotension mandates conversion regardless of the presence or absence of a detectable endoleak.

### Life expectancy after EVAR

The cumulative survival rate at 48 months for the whole cohort of patients in the EUROSTAR series was 75% [6]. In most cases, death was not directly related to the aneurysm. Schermerhorn and coworkers [11] compared life expectancy after EVAR and after open repair by using a Markov decision analysis model with data from EUROSTAR. In this model, hypothetical patients with AAA suitable for repair with either strategy were assigned to defined health states according to probabilities of success and failure, which were derived from current literature. Life expectancy was essentially the same for patients after EVAR or open repair: in a base-case analysis of 70-year-old men, life expectancy was 7 quality-adjusted life-years for patients who had EVAR and for patients who had open repair. This study was prompted by published reports in which it was suggested that operative mortality is lower after EVAR than after open repair for patients of any age. The suggestion may seem unfounded because no published trial shows a significant difference between EVAR and open repair. Schermerhorn and coworkers [11], however, concluded that the two groups of patients in this model were probably not equivalent (and thus the results may not be definitive) because patients were included who were considered to be unfit for open repair.


## Conclusion

Patients who undergo EVAR need careful long-term follow-up to detect and treat complications and to meet the ultimate goal of aneurysm repair: to prevent aneurysmal rupture. After EVAR, a considerable number of patients may need reintervention and conversion to open repair at a rate that seems to be higher than the rate for patients after open repair. Although death resulting from aneurysmal rupture after EVAR seems to be a relatively rare event, conversion to open repair is associated with considerable mortality, and this fact highlights the need for accurate definitions of the indications for conversion.


## References

1 Patel ST, Haser PB, Bush HL Jr, Kent KC. The cost-effectiveness of endovascular repair versus open surgical repair of abdominal aortic aneurysms: a decision analysis model. *J Vasc Surg* 1999; **29**: 958–72.
2 Chaikof EL, Blankensteijn JD, Harris PL et al., for the Ad Hoc Committee for Standardized Reporting Practices in Vascular Surgery of the Society for Vascular Surgery/American Association for Vascular Surgery. Reporting standards for endovascular aortic aneurysm repair. *J Vasc Surg* 2002; **35**: 1048–60.
3 White GH, Yu W, May J, Chaufour X, Stephen MS. Endoleak as a complication of endoluminal grafting of abdominal aortic aneurysms: classification, incidence, diagnosis, and management. *J Endovasc Surg* 1997; **4**: 152–68.
4 Gilling-Smith G, Brennan J, Harris P et al. Endotension after endovascular aneurysm repair: definition, classification, and strategies for surveillance and intervention. *J Endovasc Surg* 1999; **6**: 305–7.

5 Matsumura JS, Moore WS, for the Endovascular Technologies Investigators. Clinical consequences of periprosthetic leak after endovascular repair of abdominal aortic aneurysm. *J Vasc Surg* 1998; 27: 606–13.

6 Harris PL, Vallabhaneni SR, Desgranges P *et al.*, for the EUROSTAR Collaborators. Incidence and risk factors of late rupture, conversion, and death after endovascular repair of infrarenal aortic aneurysms: the EUROSTAR experience. *J Vasc Surg* 2000; 32: 739–49.

7 van Marrewijk C, Buth J, Harris PL *et al.* Significance of endoleaks after endovascular repair of abdominal aortic aneurysms: the EUROSTAR experience. *J Vasc Surg* 2002; 35: 461–73.

8 Lumsden AB, Allen RC, Chaikof EL *et al.* Delayed rupture of aortic aneurysms following endovascular stent grafting. *Am J Surg* 1995; 170: 174–8.

9 Kantonen I, Lepäntalo M, Brommels M *et al.*, and the Finnvasc Study Group. Mortality in ruptured abdominal aortic aneurysms. *Eur J Vasc Endovasc Surg* 1999; 17: 208–12.

10 Ohki T, Veith FJ, Shaw P *et al.* Increasing incidence of midterm and long-term complications after endovascular graft repair of abdominal aortic aneurysms: a note of caution based on a 9-year experience. *Ann Surg* 2001; 234: 323–34.

11 Schermerhorn ML, Finlayson SR, Fillinger MF *et al.* Life expectancy after endovascular versus open abdominal aortic aneurysm repair: results of a decision analysis model on the basis of data from EUROSTAR. *J Vasc Surg* 2002; 36: 1112–20.

CHAPTER 3

# Imaging techniques and protocols for endovascular repair of abdominal aortic aneurysms

**Ricardo Paz-Fumagalli, MD, J. Mark McKinney, MD, Andrew H. Stockland, MD**

## Introduction

Endovascular repair of abdominal aortic aneurysms (AAAs) requires accurate imaging for patient selection, device choice and sizing, and monitoring during and after repair. Imaging protocols must be implemented to provide the endovascular team with detailed morphologic information. Carefully matching the device and the vascular dimensions minimizes technical failures and delayed stent graft problems. After endovascular AAA repair, imaging studies are used to ascertain complete exclusion of the aneurysm and the integrity of the stent graft and to direct intervention (whether surgical or percutaneous) when needed.

Preoperative planning requires evaluation of the vascular dimensions, the adequacy of attachment sites, and the quality of iliofemoral access. Important dimensions include the diameters of the aortic neck, aneurysm sac, terminal aorta, and iliac arteries and the lengths of the aortic neck, infrarenal aorta, and common iliac arteries. The morphologic features of the vessel and wall determine the adequacy of the vascular sites for device attachment. The location, number, and patency of renal arteries must be noted. The infrarenal neck is examined for mural thrombi, large calcified plaques, angulation with respect to the aneurysm proper, and parallelism of the neck walls. The aneurysm is examined for tortuosity and distribution of luminal thrombi. The extent of iliac calcification, the presence of stenosis, and the location and patency of the hypogastric arteries are recorded.

## Computed tomography

Computed tomography is the primary method for preoperative and post-operative imaging for endovascular aortic stent graft procedures. Computed tomography is readily available, relatively inexpensive, reproducible, and quick. With multi-detector row computed tomography, examinations are performed in less time and with coverage of greater vascular volumes. In contradistinction to conventional angiography, volumetric acquisition by computed tomography allows vascular features to be demonstrated from any angle. Multiplanar reconstructions and three-dimensional (3D) and volumetric analyses are performed routinely with imaging workstations linked to computed tomographic (CT) imaging equipment. The main disadvantage of computed tomography is the need for iodinated contrast medium. For patients with renal insufficiency, ultrasonography (US) or magnetic resonance imaging (MRI) may be more appropriate. Noncontrast computed tomography is excellent for evaluation of aneurysm sac dimensions, but without intravenous contrast medium, its utility for detection of endoleaks is limited.

Two-phase CT scanning is performed with multi-detector hardware. The initial noncontrast scan is for documentation of vascular calcification. Scanning is performed from the dome of the diaphragm to the lower margin of the symphysis pubis. A slice thickness of 2.5 mm is used. The second contrast-enhanced phase is timed for maximal arterial enhancement. A volume of 125 mL of nonionic contrast medium is injected at a rate of 4 mL/s through an antecubital 18-gauge intravenous cannula. The postcontrast scan is usually obtained with a routine 30-s scan delay, but timing studies performed at a single level may increase the reliability of acquisition during optimal arterial enhancement [1]. Another method is to use automated triggering performed by software on the CT scanner (Figure 3.1). The postcontrast acquisition is obtained from 1 cm proximal to the celiac trunk to the lesser trochanters. Slice thickness is kept at 2.5 mm and reconstructions are performed at 2.5-mm intervals. Although other centers reconstruct at smaller intervals to provide overlapping data to improve multiplanar reconstructions, we have found that

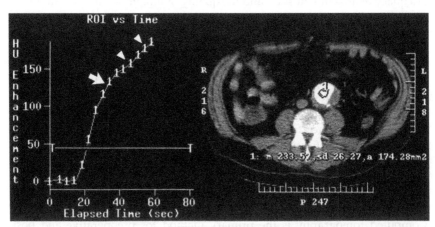

**Figure 3.1** Computed tomographic scan enhancement curve of a patient with abdominal aortic aneurysm. The region of interest (ROI) was the lumen of the aneurysm. Injection of 125 mL of nonionic contrast medium through a peripheral vein sharply increased the Hounsfield units (HU), with optimal aortic enhancement (arrow) at 30 s and a slower increase during the rest of the injection (arrowheads).

**Table 3.1** Protocol for helical computed tomographic evaluation before and after endovascular repair of abdominal aortic aneurysms.

| Variable | Precontrast | Postcontrast | |
| --- | --- | --- | --- |
| | | Arterial phase | Delayed |
| Collimation, mm | 2.5 | 2.5 | 2.5 |
| Reconstruction interval, mm | 2.5 | 2.5 | 2.5 |
| Table speed, mm/s | 15 | 15 | 15 |
| Pitch | 6 | 6 | 6 |
| Injection rate, mL/s | – | 4 | – |
| Contrast medium | – | 125 mL, nonionic | – |
| Imaging delay, s | – | 30 | 90 |

2.5-mm intervals are excellent for diagnosis and have the benefit of decreasing the number of images to view and archive. The CT scan variables are defined in Table 3.1.

The postoperative CT scan includes a precontrast acquisition of the graft only. The postcontrast scan is performed as previously described for preoperative evaluation. An additional delayed postcontrast scan at 90 s is added to the protocol for detection of delayed endoleaks [1,2]. Noncontrast images do not necessarily need to be reacquired with each new postoperative scan. Baseline noncontrast studies obtained during the preoperative evaluation and first postoperative evaluation are adequate for documentation of the vascular calcification pattern [3].

Interpretation is best accomplished on an imaging workstation. The aorta and its branches are interrogated with mouse-controlled cine viewing. For modular and adjustable stent grafts, analysis of the axial images for diameters and lengths is adequate for preoperative planning. Our practice is to report all CT aortic diameter and length measurements in a standard template (Appendix). This allows the entire endovascular team to become familiar with the pattern of measurements in the CT report.

The measurements are obtained from the axial images. Diameters are recorded as the shortest linear distance (short axis) across the lumen on the selected axial image to avoid overestimation of diameter caused by tortuosity. Orthogonal cross sections give the most accurate diameter but require having multiplanar reconstruction capability (Figure 3.2). Diameters are measured from the outer surface of the vascular wall to the outer surface of the opposite wall. This measurement method minimizes problems with anchoring the device and achieving an effective seal as a result of exuberant plaque or layered thrombus. Endovascular planning using the opacified lumen dimensions is discouraged. Lengths are calculated from simple slice location (table position) subtraction. For tortuous vessels, more accurate measurements are obtained with reconstructed 3D maximum-intensity projection CT data and 3D shaded-surface display images (CT angiography) (Figure 3.3).

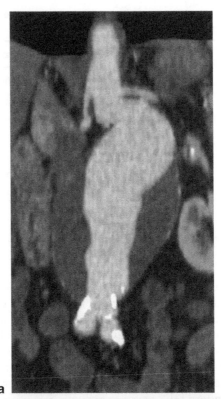

a

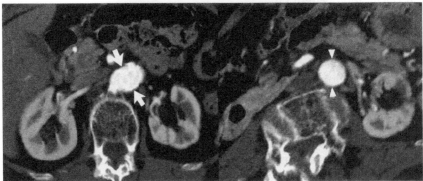

b

**Figure 3.2** Multiplanar reconstruction (MPR) of axial computed tomographic data. This method of image manipulation is useful for evaluation of the morphologic features of the infrarenal neck and its angulation in relation to the abdominal aortic aneurysm sac and for correction of tortuosity. (a) Coronal MPR of the aorta obtained from axial source images. The distance between the left renal artery and the aneurysm is extremely short, and the angle formed by the aneurysm neck and sac is acute. Endovascular repair with a stent graft is not feasible. (b) Tortuous infrarenal aortic neck. Measurement of the short axis of the infrarenal neck in the original axial image (left; arrows) usually yields comparable results to measurement of a true cross section obtained with MPR (right; arrowheads).

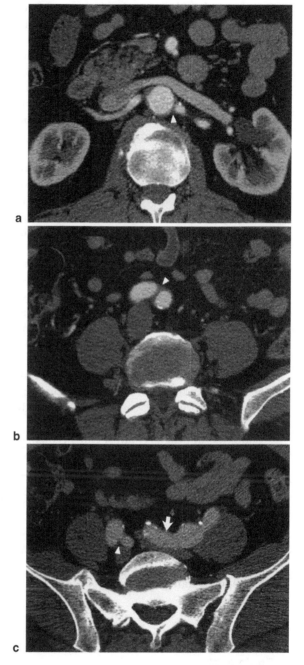

**Figure 3.3** Calculation of aortoiliac length by table position. (a) At the undersurface of the most distal renal artery (arrowhead), the table position was −170 mm. (b) At the aortic bifurcation (arrowhead), the table position was −285 mm. (c) At the right common iliac artery bifurcation (arrowhead), the table position was −315 mm. Simple subtraction provided direct longitudinal measurements in millimeters. The length from the most distal renal artery to the aortic bifurcation was 115 mm, and the length from the most distal renal artery to the right common iliac artery bifurcation was 145 mm. This measurement method is accurate in the absence of tortuosity. Multiplanar and three-dimensional reconstructions, or conventional angiography, may be needed for measurements of markedly tortuous vessels, such as the left common iliac artery (arrow).

Conventional angiography has been considered more accurate with tortuosity, but CT angiography may be the only method necessary for planning [4]. Maximum-intensity projection of the CT data is an excellent way to evaluate the calcium burden in the iliac arteries. The most accurate method to determine the diameter of vascular structures is to define a center line over the length of the vessel and to obtain diameters from orthogonal cross sections. More accurate length measurements can be obtained by measuring the center line through the vessel [5,6]. These reconstructed CT data can be obtained with dedicated workstations or sent out for commercial software planning (Figure 3.4).

Postoperative evaluation protocols are determined both by the clinical trial protocols of the manufacturers and by the experience of the local endovascular team. Synchronized cine evaluation of the previous and current studies on the imaging workstation allows direct comparison of vessel diameters and detection of endoleaks. Typically, postoperative CT follow-up is obtained at 1, 3, 6, and 12 months after implantation. Annual follow-up is routinely acquired thereafter [7]. If an endoleak is present, more frequent CT follow-up may be necessary until the sac closes spontaneously and a decrease in size is documented or until the leak is closed therapeutically.

The most reliable indicator of aneurysm sac exclusion is a progressive decrease in aneurysm sac size. Simple diameter measurement in one or two planes is relatively insensitive to overall changes in aneurysm sac size but is the easiest method and is sufficient if the diameters clearly decrease over time (Figure 3.5). Aortic sac volume measurements may provide a more reliable indicator of aneurysm exclusion, but they are time consuming, and a postprocessing workstation and dedicated software are required [5,8,9].

Endoleaks appear as contrast enhancement outside of the endograft lumen and within the aneurysm sac. Review of the noncontrast images is helpful to determine that areas of increased attenuation are contrast enhancement and not preexisting calcified plaque. Delayed images obtained 90 s after the injection of contrast medium are useful to look for delayed endoleaks that occur from vascular collateral pathways, but most endoleaks are visible during the arterial phase of the scan [1]. Computed tomography is considered the most useful tool for endoleak evaluation (Figure 3.6). The sensitivity and specificity of endoleak detection have been calculated at 92% and 90%, respectively, for computed tomography and 63% and 77%, respectively, for conventional angiography [10].

## Conventional angiography

### Equipment
Angiographic evaluation and intervention is best accomplished in a dedicated environment (conventional angiography room or endovascular suite).

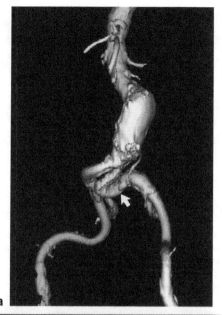

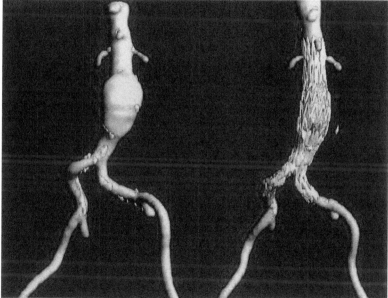

**Figure 3.4** (a) Three-dimensional (3D) surface-rendered reconstruction of axial computed tomographic (CT) data. The left common iliac artery is extremely tortuous (arrow). This type of reconstruction provides "angiographic" information that can be used for operative planning without the need for a conventional angiogram. (b) 3D reconstructions produced commercially from axial CT data show the aneurysm before (left) and after (right) stent graft placement. Commercial imaging services are an alternative to in-house image manipulation. (Courtesy of Medical Media Systems, West Lebanon, NH. By permission.)

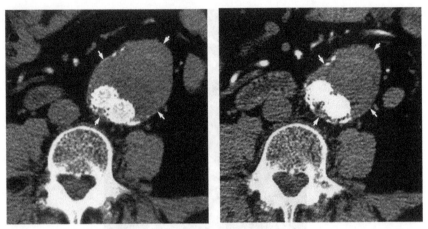

a                                                                                              b

**Figure 3.5** (a) The dimensions of the abdominal aortic aneurysm (AAA) sac (arrows) 1 month after endovascular repair are 71 × 55 mm. (b) The dimensions of the AAA sac (arrows) 11 months after repair decreased to 63 × 47 mm and the sac had visibly contracted from its original shape. Lack of sac shrinkage or enlargement may indicate failure of endovascular repair, and it most commonly occurs in the presence of an endoleak.

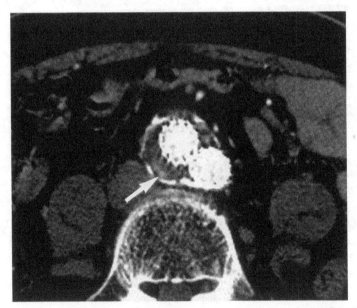

**Figure 3.6** Axial computed tomographic (CT) scan of a type II endoleak from lumbar collaterals. Note the subtle enhancement in the aortic sac (arrow). Many endoleaks are readily visible on CT scans.

Intraprocedural angiography is adequate in an operating room adapted for endovascular procedures with a C-arm, but a specially designed endovascular suite that meets operating room standards provides optimal quality with the greatest flexibility and capabilities [11]. The operating room C-arm has a smaller image intensifier, a smaller range of motion and angulation, and less beam collimation capability, and it requires a radiolucent operating table. When procedures are done in the operating room, the radiation dose to the patient and operators is usually greater. Ideally, the equipment has free-floating table capability and variable height. High-quality digital imaging ($1024 \times 1024$ matrix) provides instant acquisition and display. Features that are standard in dedicated angiographic equipment but not in operating room C-arms include variable frame rates, magnification, road mapping, fluoro fade, photo file, electronic archiving, and postprocessing of images (contrast and edge enhancement, variable display level and window, pixel shifting, pan and zoom, vessel sizing, and calculation of percentage stenosis) [12]. Digital subtraction angiography helps decrease the required volume of iodinated contrast medium and permits imaging with carbon dioxide [12]. It is adversely affected by motion, but unsubtracted imaging can be diagnostic. Table 3.2 lists supplies needed for angiography.

## Preoperative angiography

A common femoral artery is catheterized percutaneously with a 5F or 6F hemostatic sheath. A 4F, 5F, or 6F pigtail catheter is most commonly used for abdominal aortography. The pigtail catheter is positioned just above the renal arteries in the anteroposterior projection and above the celiac artery in the lateral projection. Contrast medium is injected at a rate of 15–20 mL/s for a total of 30–40 mL. Bilateral 25–30° oblique pelvic angiograms are obtained with the catheter positioned in the terminal aorta and contrast medium injected at a rate of 7–10 mL/s for a total of 15–20 mL. Nonionic contrast media are recommended because of their lesser toxicity and greater patient comfort. Imaging should be carried out at 1–2 frames/s. For measurement, a 20-cm graduated pigtail catheter is practical because lengths can be determined quickly by counting markers and it also serves as a reference for calibration of electronic calipers without having to correct for a magnification factor (Figure 3.7).

Preoperative angiography can delineate the morphologic features of the aneurysm, the infrarenal neck, and the access iliac vessels. It has the advantage of displaying the luminal morphologic features of long vascular segments, but conventional angiography alone is inadequate for device sizing and selection for several reasons. It underestimates diameters, it does not measure the length of the neck accurately, and it does not detail the characteristics of plaque, thrombus, and calcification in the aortic neck or iliac arteries. Parallax and foreshortening are additional problems [13]. Conventional angiographic measurements of length are accurate but not routinely indicated because they closely correlate with CT angiographic measurements

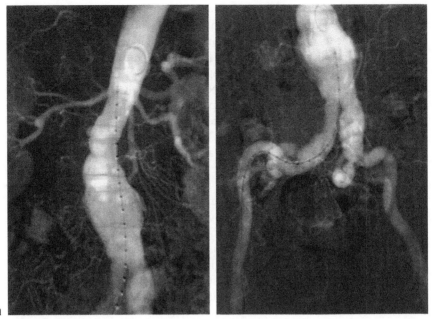

a

b

**Figure 3.7** Preoperative conventional angiogram of aortoiliac vessels. The use of a graduated-marker catheter provides a practical way to measure length, particularly when the vessels are tortuous. In the absence of tortuosity, most patients do not need a preoperative angiogram, and a computed tomographic scan will suffice for procedural planning. (a) Measurement of the aorta from the renal arteries to the bifurcation. (b) Measurement of the common iliac arteries from the origin to the bifurcation.

of the length from the most distal renal artery to the aortic bifurcation and the length of the common iliac arteries [14]. Although some authors have suggested that neither CT scanning nor conventional angiography alone is sufficient for preoperative planning [15], in our practice preoperative angiography is limited to selected patients, such as those who require preoperative coil embolization of the hypogastric artery or stenting of the renal artery or those who have tortuous iliac arteries. Proper planning does not require the use of invasive imaging. In a series of 25 patients studied with spiral computed tomography and 3D reconstructions and without conventional angiography, all patients received endografts as planned without graft-related complications [6]. Conventional angiography is recommended during the initial experience for correlation with cross-sectional imaging because iliac tortuosity can make measurements of length difficult with computed tomography. After the operator gains confidence interpreting cross-sectional imaging, a shift to selective, rather than routine, angiography helps minimize costs and morbidity.

**Table 3.2** Basic angiographic supplies.

| Item | Description | Purpose |
|------|-------------|---------|
| Power injector | Free standing; table or ceiling mounted | High-contrast volume/rate injections |
| Injector syringes | 150 mL | – |
| Pressure transducer | – | Evaluation for flow-limiting lesions |
| Contrast medium | Nonionic, preferably iso-osmolar | Less toxicity |
| Entry needle | Seldinger or open end: 19 gauge, 18 gauge | Initial arterial puncture |
| Guidewires | Bentson: 0.035 inch, 145 cm, 260 cm | Initial access; basic selective catheterization; catheter exchanges |
| | J wire: 0.035 inch, 145 cm | Initial access |
| | Hydrophilic: angled, 0.035 inch, 180 cm | Traversal of stenoses and selective catheterization |
| Torque device | 0.038 inch, 0.018 inch | Steering of guidewires for selective catheterization |
| Fascial dilators | 5F, 6F | To facilitate introduction of catheters and sheaths |
| Sheaths | Hemostatic valve: 5F, 6F | To facilitate introduction of catheters, catheter exchanges, and selective catheterization |
| Catheters | Pigtail: 4F, 5F, 6F | Basic aortography |
| | Graduated marker pigtail: 5F, 6F | Preoperative and intraoperative selection of device length |
| | Various angled catheters (vertebral, Kumpe, multipurpose): 5F | Selective catheterization |
| | H1H: 5F | Selective catheterization |
| | Cobra shaped: 5F | Selective catheterization |
| | Various reversed curves (visceral, selective, Sos, Simmons 1): 5F | Visceral or hypogastric selective catheterization; catheterization over stent graft bifurcation |
| | Coaxial microcatheters: 3F | Superselective catheterization and coil embolization |
| Syringes | 10 mL, 20 mL | Saline flushing and hand injection of contrast medium |
| | 60 mL | Access sheath aspiration during completion aortogram |
| Stopcocks | 3-way | Continuous catheter flushing; pressure transduction; port for injections of contrast medium |
| Flow switch | – | Hemostasis at catheter hub |

## Intraoperative angiography

Intraoperative conventional angiography and fluoroscopy are unrivaled for guiding the successful deployment of aortic stent grafts, offering fast and reliable localization of the renal arteries and aortic and iliac bifurcations and evaluation of aneurysm exclusion. Intraprocedural use of a graduated-marker catheter helps confirm the appropriate choice of device dimensions. A pigtail catheter is introduced through a sheath in the common femoral artery contralateral to the site of device insertion and is placed just proximal to the renal arteries. To minimize exposure to contrast medium, the renal arteries can be localized with short bursts of small volumes of contrast medium (10 mL at 30 mL/s from the power injector) and imaging at 2–4 frames/s (Figure 3.8).

The exact location of the most distal renal artery can be marked by several means. Road-map and fluoro-fade functions, an outline of the artery on the fluoroscopy monitor with a dry-erase marker, placement of stickers with radiopaque markers over the patient's abdomen, boards with sliding markers, and bone landmarks can be used, but they are all susceptible to parallax if the table is moved after acquisition of the angiogram.

Because the stent graft can be deployed alongside the catheter, additional angiograms are possible after deployment, but the catheter must be removed when use of the access site is required, such as during cannulation of the con-

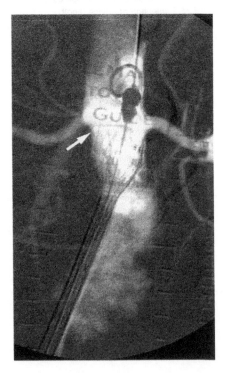

**Figure 3.8** Intraoperative aortogram during stent graft deployment confirms the exact location of the renal arteries and positioning of the stent graft (arrow) distal to the most distal renal artery. If the device compromises the renal artery ostium, the device can be repositioned before it is fully deployed.

tralateral limb gate and placement of the contralateral limb extension of a modular device. Some operators place the pigtail catheter through an arterial puncture separate from the arterial access sheath, allowing them to keep the pigtail catheter in place for the entire procedure. Hand-injection angiography can be done to confirm proper cannulation of the contralateral limb gate of a modular device, and hand-injection retrograde angiography through the access sheaths is ideal for localization of iliac bifurcations. After complete device deployment, aortography that encompasses the length from the suprarenal aorta to the external iliac arteries is done with a larger volume of contrast medium, 30–40 mL, at a rate of 20–30 mL/s with imaging at 2–4 frames/s. The completion angiogram shows the final configuration of the device, its relationship with the renal and hypogastric arteries, and the complete exclusion of the aneurysm. Because the sheaths frequently obstruct flow, brisk aspiration of the access sheaths with 60-mL syringes during completion aortography creates a "runoff" effect. Failure to perform this maneuver produces an angiogram that lacks diagnostic quality, especially if the hypogastric arteries are occluded or severely stenotic.

Because angiography can be carried out to the capillary and venous phases of flow, endoleaks that appear late in the timing sequence can be detected. CT scanning is more sensitive to endoleaks but cannot be used during the procedure. The main limitation of angiography is its relative insensitivity to incomplete stent apposition to the arterial wall, kinks, and narrowing or folding of the device. If these problems are suspected after balloon dilatation of all landing sites and device joints and limbs, intravascular ultrasonography (IVUS) may offer more detailed information. IVUS was found to have a sensitivity of 92%, as compared with 50% for conventional angiography, in evaluating vascular stenosis [16]. Intraprocedural pressure gradients can be measured, but one should exercise caution in interpreting the measurements because occlusion of the femoral arteries by the large sheaths and vessel loops may mask significant gradients.

## Postoperative angiography

Routine postprocedure angiography is unnecessary. It should be reserved for patients with problems such as device migration, kinks or stenosis, and endoleaks that require treatment. In a comparison between CT and conventional angiography, the sensitivity and specificity of CT angiography for endoleak were 92% and 90%, respectively, and for conventional angiography, 63% and 77%, respectively [10]. Angiography can be used to confirm the cause of endoleaks and the exact flow patterns into and out of the aortic sac. After problems are correctly diagnosed, angiography can be used to guide treatment, including balloon dilation, stent placement, placement of additional stent grafts for extension of the proximal or distal landing sites, and obliteration of endoleaks. The angiographic evaluation is always started with an aortogram, but methodical selective angiography with various diagnostic and guiding catheters and microcatheters may be needed. Some type I and type

III endoleaks are difficult to pinpoint. In some cases it may be necessary to probe the attachment sites and device junctions with the tip of the catheter or to perform either selective angiography of each limb with or without balloon occlusion or retrograde iliac angiography [17]. Type II endoleaks may be complex, with contributing collaterals arising from the inferior mesenteric, lumbar, and hypogastric vessels. Typically, angiograms show certain vessels providing the inflow into the endoleaks and others providing the outflow. Such a circuit is necessary to keep the endoleak active. Evaluation of type II endoleaks begins with an abdominal aortogram. Selective hypogastric and superior mesenteric artery angiograms are required (Figure 3.9). Angiographic obliteration of a type II endoleak may be formidable, requiring an experienced interventionalist and a fully equipped angiography suite stocked with various microcatheters and microcoils. Description of the superselective coil embolization procedure, or direct sac puncture, is beyond the scope of this chapter.

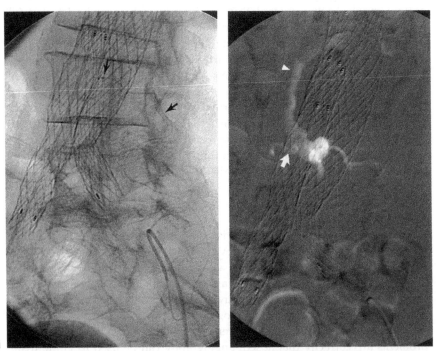

a                                                                                                                                      b

**Figure 3.9** Superselective angiography of a type II endoleak. (a) A microcatheter was placed into the aortic sac via the left fourth lumbar artery; catheterization was through a left iliolumbar collateral arising from the left hypogastric artery (arrows). (b) Angiogram of the aortic sac demonstrated the other lumbar artery forming part of the endoleak circuit (arrow) and contrast medium (arrowhead) extending into the aortic sac. Superselective catheterization permitted closure of the endoleak with embolization agents.

## Magnetic resonance imaging

MRI is an alternative to CT scanning in the preoperative and postoperative evaluation for endovascular repair of AAAs. It is particularly useful if the patient is at risk for nephrotoxicity from iodinated contrast medium or has a documented, potentially life-threatening allergy. MRI is not appropriate for patients with cardiac pacemakers, a history of metallic fragments or foreign bodies in the eye, or non-MRI-compatible implants for safety reasons or because of substantial image artifact (such as from implanted vascular stents). Postoperatively, MRI is used to demonstrate endoleaks, particularly with stent grafts constructed with nitinol wire [18]. Ferromagnetic stent grafts, such as those built with Gianturco Z stents (Cook, Inc, Bloomington, IN), severely limit the usefulness of MRI because of magnetic susceptibility artifact. Problems arise when MRI is to be used with patients who cannot hold their breath or who are claustrophobic. Although MRI cannot be used to demonstrate the extent of vascular calcification, nonenhanced computed tomography can.

In a study of 61 patients that compared magnetic resonance angiography, CT angiography, and conventional angiography, magnetic resonance angiography was found to provide all the relevant information for preoperative planning [19]. T2-weighted axial images show the aortic diameters and extent of the aneurysm, the features of mural thrombus, perianeurysmal inflammatory changes or signs of rupture, and anatomical variants, such as a retroaortic left renal vein. Gadolinium-enhanced 3D magnetic resonance angiography demonstrates the aortoiliac lumen, length and tortuosity, and the number, location, and atherosclerotic disease of visceral vessels. If obtained, delayed acquisitions produce an abdominal venogram. Multiplanar reformatted images provide the diameter and length measurements necessary for device selection. Neschis et al. [20] studied 96 patients who had contrast-medium allergy or creatinine levels >1.5 mg/dL and who were evaluated preoperatively with MRI. These patients were compared with a group evaluated with computed tomography. There were no differences in intraoperative access failure, use of stent graft extensions, surgical conversions, or fluoroscopy and procedure times. Postoperatively, these authors found no statistical difference in detection of endoleaks, but a direct comparison of MRI and computed tomography was not carried out.

Because MRI protocols and the imaging needs of endovascular aortic intervention are constantly changing, cooperation is necessary between magnetic resonance and vascular/interventional radiologists. Although technical details serve as a guide (Table 3.3), they are subject to modifications demanded by changes in medical practice and technologic advances. MRI is carried out with the body coil, but an anteroposterior phased-array surface coil improves the signal-to-noise ratio. Inspiratory breath-hold imaging is ideal. If tolerated, aliasing artifact can be decreased if the patient's arms are positioned above the head. Gadolinium is infused through an antecubital vein at a rate of 1–3 mL/s for a volume of 40 mL. Automated bolus timing soft-

**Table 3.3** Magnetic resonance angiography features for evaluation of abdominal aortic aneurysms at Mayo Clinic in Jacksonville, Florida.

| Feature | Technical detail |
|---|---|
| Equipment | Siemens Symphony with 1.5 T MRease platform* |
| Sequence | Flash 3D* |
| Plane | Coronal |
| Field of view | 36 cm |
| Slice thickness | 1.5 mm |
| Distance factor (gap) | 20% |
| Slices per slab | 52; 1 group |
| Phase | Right to left |
| TR | 4.53 ms |
| TE | 1.54 ms |
| Flip angle | 25° |
| Bandwidth | 390 Hz per pixel |
| Fat saturation | Applied |
| Matrix | 256 × 225 |
| Fourier | 6/8 partial |
| Scan time | 25 s |
| Breath-hold | Yes |
| Timing gadolinium bolus | 2–3 mL |
| Volume of contrast medium | 35 mL |
| Contrast medium injection rate | 2 mL/s |
| Reconstructions | Maximum-intensity projection, multiplanar |

*Siemens AG, Munich, Germany.

ware is helpful for imaging during the period of most intense enhancement, especially for patients with cardiac dysfunction. T2-weighted axial images and 3D time-of-flight gadolinium-enhanced angiography in the coronal plane are acquired. The 3D data can be reformatted in the axial plane (which is helpful for endoleak evaluation) and displayed as a maximum-intensity projection 3D reconstruction. T1-weighted axial precontrast images help in distinguishing gadolinium enhancement of an endoleak from hyperintense methemoglobin within the thrombosed aortic sac (Figure 3.10) [18].

## Intravascular ultrasonography

Miniaturized ultrasound transducers are mounted on catheters and placed inside the vascular lumen to image the vascular wall and lumen with high resolution. IVUS is based on the same principles as general diagnostic US but with the added advantage that the close proximity to the vessel wall allows imaging with higher frequencies. IVUS provides measurements of vascular diameter and length and evaluation of vascular anatomical and pathologic features. In patients with AAA, IVUS has been used during the preoperative

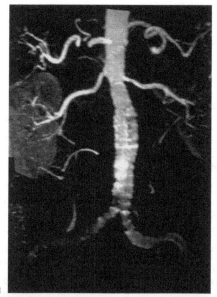

a

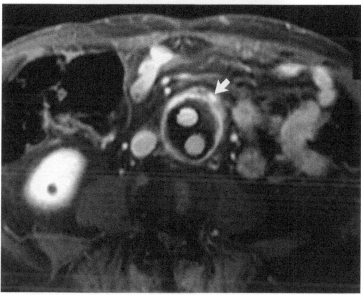

b

**Figure 3.10** Magnetic resonance imaging of an abdominal aortic aneurysm treated with a bifurcated stent graft. (a) Gadolinium-enhanced magnetic resonance angiogram demonstrates preservation of the renal arteries and patency of the stent graft limbs. The scalloped appearance of the image is caused by metallic artifact from the stents; metallic artifact is remarkably minimal if the stents are made of nonferromagnetic alloys. Stainless steel stents produce more artifact that severely degrades the images. (b) Gadolinium-enhanced T1-weighted axial image of the repaired aorta, obtained with fat suppression. Lack of enhancement within the aortic sac thrombus excludes an endoleak. The lumina of the stent graft limbs enhance normally. The intense enhancement of the aortic wall (arrow) is caused by gadolinium uptake from an earlier injection of contrast medium. (Courtesy of Scott Erickson, MD; Milwaukee, WI. By permission.)

evaluation to direct aortic stent graft placement and after deployment to evaluate the final result [21,22]. Unlike other cross-sectional imaging techniques, IVUS can be used during the endovascular procedure, decreasing fluoroscopy time and use of iodinated contrast material.

## Equipment

Two types of intravascular transducers are available, mechanical and phased array. Both can be used successfully for planning and evaluating aortic stent grafting. The mechanical type has an element that is rotated by a shaft controlled by a motor drive. The rotation generates images of the entire circumference of the vessel. This system has a monorail configuration over a guidewire, which decreases catheter pushability and trackability. The second type, which we use in our practice, consists of an array of 64 elements that transmit electronic information in sequence, generating a circumferential image. This type has no moving parts and is truly coaxial, the wire traversing the entire catheter length. This design improves trackability and pushability. For aortic applications, we use an 8.2F transducer that has a frequency of 10 MHz, requires a 9F sheath, and images sections up to 6 cm in diameter.

## Anatomy

The three layers of normal arteries are recognizable with IVUS. The intima and adventitia are hyperechoic, separated by the hypoechoic media. However, these layers may not be readily visible in large elastic arteries, such as the aorta. Alterations of this pattern can be caused by atherosclerosis or by the presence of intravascular devices such as guidewires, catheters, sheaths, stents, and graft material. Plaque thickens the intima and, when calcified, causes bright echoes and acoustic shadowing. Ulceration and other morphologic changes can be visualized clearly. Arterial branches appear as anechoic gaps in the vessel wall [23].

## Technique

During the examination, identification of the celiac, superior mesenteric, renal, and iliac arteries and the left renal vein allows proper orientation. Generally IVUS provides images perpendicular to the vessel lumen for accurate diameter measurement, but in large and tortuous vessels the IVUS catheter may not be aligned parallel to the lumen, so that the cross sections may be oblique. In this case, the short axis of the oval image of the vessel provides the more accurate measurement.

Length measurements can be acquired during withdrawal of the IVUS catheter, but first the slack that builds up during introduction of the catheter must be eliminated. The length of catheter withdrawn from the sheath reflects the distance traveled from one landmark to another, such as from the most distal renal artery to the iliac bifurcation [21]. This measurement closely approximates the shortest distance from one point to another, but this is not necessarily the path that the stent graft follows. Such measurements tend to underestimate the ideal device length by a mean of 15 mm [24].

## Applications

Preoperatively, IVUS can be combined with angiography to obtain vascular diameters and lengths [22]. In our practice we do not do this routinely because helical computed tomography has largely replaced angiography. A clear indication would be needed to justify the additional procedure and expense. Some differences can be demonstrated between measurements obtained with IVUS and CT angiography or conventional angiography, but generally, these small discrepancies are of little practical importance because device lengths are determined in centimeters. The modular nature of many devices allows for intraprocedural adjustments of length [25].

During aortic stent graft placement, IVUS can be used to determine appropriate lengths and diameters of the device components and to select sites for device placement. IVUS does not entirely eliminate intraprocedural angiography because IVUS may fail to demonstrate accessory renal arteries, although an excellent correlation with conventional angiography has been shown [25,26]. Real-time monitoring of the device deployment is an appealing application, but it has not been consistently reliable [26].

After endovascular repair of an AAA, IVUS can be used to demonstrate problems with full apposition of the stents with the aortic and iliac walls and full expansion of the stents, which predisposes to endoleaks or limb thrombosis (Figure 3.11). Kinks, folds, or other abnormalities that decrease the size of the vascular lumen are best evaluated with IVUS. For evaluating vascular stenoses, IVUS was found to have a sensitivity of 92% as compared with 50% for conventional angiography [16]. Extensive artifact from the stents, however, precludes visualization of the adjacent arterial wall. Devices with

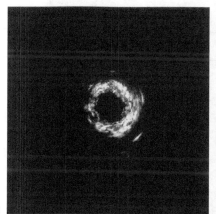
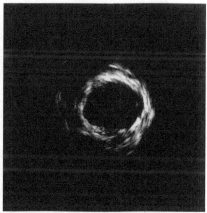

a                                                                                           b

**Figure 3.11** Intravascular ultrasonography during endovascular repair of an abdominal aortic aneurysm with a bifurcated stent graft. (a) Cross-sectional image of an incompletely expanded iliac limb of the stent graft. (b) Full expansion of the limb after dilation with an angioplasty balloon. Small iliac arteries, atherosclerotic stenosis, and a narrow aortic bifurcation compromise the stent graft lumen. Full dilatation may require high pressure that cannot be generated with the compliant balloons typically used to anchor the device attachment sites and joints.

larger spaces between metallic struts allow better evaluation of stent graft placement and its relationship with the arterial wall [21,26].

## Ultrasonography

US is useful for determining and monitoring the size of an AAA, but it is of little value in the preoperative planning of endovascular repair. In the postoperative period it is an appealing alternative to computed tomography and angiography for patients who cannot receive iodinated contrast media for detecting endoleaks and monitoring sac size, two important objectives of surveillance. The value of US as a noninvasive, economical tool for detection of endoleaks is evolving (Figure 3.12). In our experience conventional US has a low sensitivity and frequently is technically inadequate for reasons such as excessive bowel gas. In a comparison of transabdominal US and contrast-enhanced computed tomography for endoleaks, US had 97% sensitivity, 74% specificity, a positive predictive value of 66%, and a negative predictive value of 98%, but a substantial number of studies had technical problems [27]. Sonographic contrast media increase the reliability and sensitivity. In a study of 18 patients with endovascular repair of AAA, conventional transabdominal US

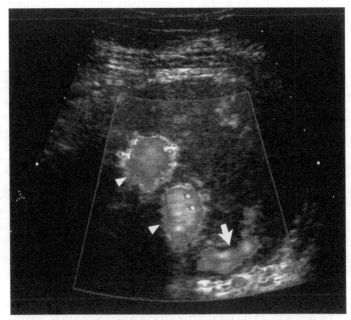

**Figure 3.12** Color Doppler imaging of the abdominal aorta after endovascular repair of an abdominal aortic aneurysm. Abnormal flow within the aortic sac (arrow), but outside of the limbs of the device (arrowheads), indicates an endoleak.

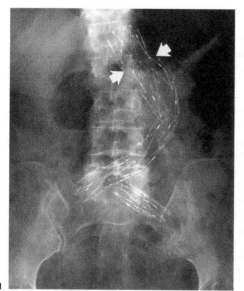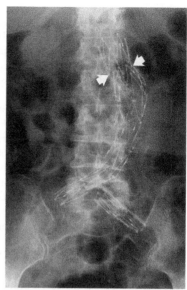

a          b

**Figure 3.13** Plain radiographs of the abdomen showing repair of an abdominal aortic aneurysm with a custom-made aortomonoiliac stent graft, a left common iliac artery occluder, and a femoral-femoral bypass graft. (a) Original position of the metallic stents (arrows). (b) Position of the metallic stents 6 months later. Separation of the stents and minimal distal migration of the device have occurred (arrows). Subtle changes can be impossible to appreciate with computed tomography, ultrasonography, or magnetic resonance imaging.

and contrast-enhanced US were compared. Without sonographic contrast medium, the sensitivity to endoleaks was 33%. With contrast medium, all endoleaks were identified. Interestingly, the investigators detected endoleaks not apparent on helical computed tomography and suggested that enhanced US may be more reliable than computed tomography [28]. Contrast-enhanced US seemed to be especially sensitive for type II leaks [29]. US is also capable of confirming limb patency but is unable to detect subtle loss of integrity of the endograft, such as metal strut breaks or migration.

## Plain radiography

Detection of a subtle loss of stent graft integrity or migration often is possible only with plain radiographs [30]. Breakage of metal struts, separation of stent links, and kinks can be impossible to detect with computed tomography or US. Clinical trial protocols of endovascular repair of AAAs require abdominal plain radiographs in different positions and obliquities, but even outside of clinical trials such images must be obtained with each follow-up CT scan and scrutinized carefully (Figure 3.13).

# References

1 Golzarian J, Dussaussois L, Abada HT *et al.* Helical CT of aorta after endoluminal stent-graft therapy: value of biphasic acquisition. *AJR Am J Roentgenol* 1998; **171**: 329–31.

2 Schurink GW, Aarts NJ, Wilde J *et al.* Endoleakage after stent-graft treatment of abdominal aneurysm: implications on pressure and imaging – an in vitro study. *J Vasc Surg* 1998; **28**: 234–41.

3 Rubin GD. Techniques for performing multidetector-row computed tomographic angiography. *Tech Vasc Interv Radiol* 2001; **4**: 2–14.

4 Broeders IA, Blankensteijn JD. Preoperative imaging of the aortoiliac anatomy in endovascular aneurysm surgery. *Semin Vasc Surg* 1999; **12**: 306–14.

5 Rubin GD, Paik DS, Johnston PC, Napel S. Measurement of the aorta and its branches with helical CT. *Radiology* 1998; **206**: 823–9.

6 Beebe HG, Kritpracha B, Serres S *et al.* Endograft planning without preoperative arteriography: a clinical feasibility study. *J Endovasc Ther* 2000; **7**: 8–15.

7 Kalman PG, Rappaport DC, Merchant N, Clarke K, Johnston KW. The value of late computed tomographic scanning in identification of vascular abnormalities after abdominal aortic aneurysm repair. *J Vasc Surg* 1999; **29**: 442–50.

8 Wever JJ, Blankensteijn JD, Th M Mali WP, Eikelboom BC. Maximal aneurysm diameter follow-up is inadequate after endovascular abdominal aortic aneurysm repair. *Eur J Vasc Endovasc Surg* 2000; **20**: 177–82.

9 Singh-Ranger R, McArthur T, Corte MD, Lees W, Adiseshiah M. The abdominal aortic aneurysm sac after endoluminal exclusion: a medium-term morphologic follow-up based on volumetric technology. *J Vasc Surg* 2000; **31**: 490–500.

10 Armerding MD, Rubin GD, Beaulieu CF *et al.* Aortic aneurismal disease: assessment of stent-graft treatment-CT versus conventional angiography. *Radiology* 2000; **215**: 138–46.

11 Katzen BT, Becker GJ, Mascioli CA *et al.* Creation of a modified angiography (endovascular) suite for transluminal endograft placement and combined interventional-surgical procedures. *J Vasc Interv Radiol* 1996; **7**: 161–7.

12 Katzen BT. Current status of digital angiography in vascular imaging. *Radiol Clin North Am* 1995; **33**: 1–14.

13 Beebe HG, Jackson T, Pigott JP. Aortic aneurysm morphology for planning endovascular aortic grafts: limitations of conventional imaging methods. *J Endovasc Surg* 1995; **2**: 139–48.

14 Broeders IA, Blankensteijn JD, Olree M, Mali W, Eikelboom BC. Preoperative sizing of grafts for transfemoral endovascular aneurysm management: a prospective comparative study of spiral CT angiography, arteriography, and conventional CT imaging. *J Endovasc Surg* 1997; **4**: 252–61.

15 Resch T, Ivancev K, Lindh M *et al.* Abdominal aortic aneurysm morphology in candidates for endovascular repair evaluated with spiral computed tomography and digital subtraction angiography. *J Endovasc Surg* 1999; **6**: 227–32.

16 Lyon RT, Veith FJ, Berdejo GL *et al.* Utility of intravascular ultrasound for assessment of endovascular procedures. Proceedings of the Joint Annual Meeting of the Society for Vascular Surgery and the International Society for Cardiovascular Surgery, North American Chapter, Boston, Massachusetts, 1–4 June 1997.

17 Matsumura JS, Ryu RK, Ouriel K. Identification and implications of transgraft microleaks after endovascular repair of aortic aneurysms. *J Vasc Surg* 2001; **34**: 190–7.

18 Engellau L, Larsson EM, Albrechtsson U, Jonung T, Ribbe E, Thorne J *et al.* Magnetic resonance imaging and MR angiography of endoluminally treated abdominal aortic aneurysms. *Eur J Vasc Endovasc Surg* 1998; **15**: 212–19.

19 Thurnher SA, Dorffner R, Thurnher MM *et al*. Evaluation of abdominal aortic aneurysm for stent-graft placement: comparison of gadolinium-enhanced MR angiography versus helical CT angiography and digital subtraction angiography. *Radiology* 1997; 205: 341–52.

20 Neschis DG, Velazquez OC, Baum RA *et al*. The role of magnetic resonance angiography for endoprosthetic design. *J Vasc Surg* 2001; 33: 488–94.

21 White RA, Donayre C, Kopchok G *et al*. Intravascular ultrasound: the ultimate tool for abdominal aortic aneurysm assessment and endovascular graft delivery. *J Endovasc Surg* 1997; 4: 45–55.

22 Levitin A. Intravascular ultrasound. *Tech Vasc Interv Radiol* 2001; 4: 66–74.

23 van Essen JA, van der Lugt A, Gussenhoven EJ *et al*. Intravascular ultrasonography allows accurate assessment of abdominal aortic aneurysm: an in vitro validation study. *J Vasc Surg* 1998; 27: 347–53.

24 Tillich M, Hill BB, Paik DS *et al*. Prediction of aortoiliac stent-graft length: comparison of measurement methods. *Radiology* 2001; 220: 475–83.

25 van Essen JA, Gussenhoven EJ, van der Lugt A *et al*. Accurate assessment of abdominal aortic aneurysm with intravascular ultrasound scanning: validation with computed tomographic angiography. *J Vasc Surg* 1999; 29: 631–8.

26 Vogt KC, Brunkwall J, Malina M *et al*. The use of intravascular ultrasound as control procedure for the deployment of endovascular stented grafts. *Eur J Vasc Endovasc Surg* 1997; 13: 592–6.

27 Sato DT, Goff CD, Gregory RT *et al*. Endoleak after aortic stent graft repair: diagnosis by color duplex ultrasound scan versus computed tomography scan. *J Vasc Surg* 1998; 28: 657–63.

28 McWilliams RG, Martin J, White D *et al*. Use of contrast-enhanced ultrasound in follow-up after endovascular aortic aneurysm repair. *J Vasc Interv Radiol* 1999; 10: 1107–14.

29 Heilberger P, Schunn C, Ritter W, Weber S, Raithel D. Postoperative color flow duplex scanning in aortic endografting. *J Endovasc Surg* 1997; 4: 262–71.

30 Moore WS, Rutherford RB, for the EVT Investigators. Transfemoral endovascular repair of abdominal aortic aneurysm: results of the North American EVT phase 1 trial. *J Vasc Surg* 1996; 23: 543–53.

## Appendix. Sample dictation template for reporting aortic measurements from computed tomography

The suprarenal aortic diameter is __ mm (D1). The interrenal aortic diameter is __ mm (D2a). The mid-proximal aortic neck diameter is __ mm (D2b). The aortic neck diameter adjacent to the aneurysm is __ mm (D2c). The maximal aortic aneurysm diameter is __ mm (D3). The terminal aortic diameter is __ mm (D4). The right common iliac artery diameter is __ mm (D5a). The left common iliac artery diameter is __ mm (D5b). The right external iliac artery diameter is __ mm (D6). The left external iliac artery diameter is __ mm (D7). The length of the aortic neck is __ mm (L1). The length of the aorta from the renal arteries to the distal aneurysms is __ mm (L2). The distance from the renal arteries to the aortic bifurcation is __ mm (L3). The distance from the most distal renal artery to the right iliac artery bifurcation is __ mm (L4a). The distance from the most distal renal artery to the left iliac artery bifurcation is __ mm (L4b).

# CHAPTER 4

# Essential operating room equipment, personnel, and catheter inventory for endovascular repair of abdominal aortic aneurysms

Peter A. Schneider, MD, Michael T. Caps, MD, MPH

## Introduction

Successful initiation of a program for endovascular repair of abdominal aortic aneurysms (AAAs) includes preparing the team and the operating room so that success may be achieved with the first case. Supplies should be procured well before the time they are needed, and arrangements must be made to purchase or lease the appropriate equipment. Each member of the endovascular team must be trained, which may include observing other teams in action and receiving in-service training. The principals in this therapeutic venture should form a plan of action and involve appropriate individuals, including operating room administrators, hospital administrators, operating room nurses, scrub nurses and circulating nurses, purchasers of the supplies and equipment, representatives from the stent graft company, the team of physicians (including physicians with experience in both open and endovascular treatment), and anesthesia personnel. The team must become familiar with the equipment, where it is located within the facility, and how the inventory is to be managed. The equipment should be stored separately from equipment for other procedures; a cart, which includes guidewires, catheters, and other accessories, is recommended for storage between cases and for use in the operating room.

Before the first case, all involved personnel should participate in a dress rehearsal and review an inventory checklist of supplies to make sure that the logistics of imaging, the injection of contrast medium, and the availability of supplies have been arranged. Contingency plans should be made in case the device fails or part of the system fails. The criteria for conversion to open repair of AAAs should be discussed and specifically enumerated before the procedure. The fully developed action plan, which is best coordinated by the team leader, also includes dates, funding sources, and costs. Endovascular AAA repair is a multistep process. Any step may be thwarted by failure to procure or deploy the appropriate supplies. Inadequacy of imaging and poor preparation of personnel are other potential reasons for failure.

Several stent grafts have been approved by the US Food and Drug Administration (FDA) for treatment of AAA: the Ancure device (Guidant Corp., Menlo Park, CA), the AneuRx device (Medtronic, Inc., Minneapolis, MN), the Excluder bifurcated endoprosthesis (W. L. Gore and Associates, Inc., Flagstaff, AZ), and the Zenith AAA endovascular graft (Cook, Inc., Bloomington, IN). This chapter focuses on the personnel, equipment, and inventory required to place these grafts. Several other grafts are in various stages of development and may have other requirements when they become clinically useful [1].

## Personnel involved in endovascular repair of abdominal aortic aneurysms

### Physicians

The physicians involved in endovascular repair of AAAs should have expertise in both open repair of vascular lesions and endovascular intervention (Table 4.1). If these skills are distributed through more than one department within an institution, an interdepartmental team of physicians is required. These physicians should have participated in the FDA-mandated training courses sponsored by the companies that distribute the repair devices. Before the procedure, the physicians should review the radiographs and make plans together.

### Scrub nurse

The scrub nurses must have experience and knowledge related to the passage of guidewires and catheters and the open repair of vascular lesions. Scrub nurses should learn the differences between the catheters and how to handle them before the first procedure. The basic concepts and skills are not intuitive and must be taught. They include, but are not limited to, the following: flushing and wiping all endovascular devices; turning all stopcocks to the "off" position; advancing or withdrawing a catheter over a guidewire while keeping the guidewire stationary; replacing guidewires into holding canisters; holding guidewires and catheters near the tip for ease of loading onto the guidewire; always keeping heparin-saline flush solution available; soaking wet gauze or nonstick bandages; partially filling syringes; and understanding radiation safety. Scrub nurses should observe other endovascular

Table 4.1 Personnel involved in endovascular repair of abdominal aortic aneurysms.

Physician experienced in both open and endovascular techniques
Scrub nurse with endovascular expertise
Circulating nurse
Radiographic technologist
Injector personnel
Company representative

procedures that are appropriate for the angiographic suite or the operating room where catheters and guidewires are being placed.

## Circulating nurse

Circulating nurses must understand the differences between various inventory items and know their specific locations. The circulating nurses must confirm that the selected package is the correct one before opening it. This is especially important for endovascular AAA repair because each stent graft component is expensive and a replacement may not be readily available. The circulating nurse must understand the sometimes subtle differences among the endovascular accessories.

## Injector personnel

An automated power injector is required for the procedure, and a person who is skilled in its function must be in the operating room. Either the circulating nurse or the radiographic technologist should be able to load and use the automated injector.

## Radiographic technologist

The radiographic technologist should have experience in vascular cases, either in the operating room or in the angiographic suite. This individual must be able to work where a sterile environment is required and where strict rules of sterility are followed. In most institutions, there is substantial variability in the experience and ability of the radiographic technologist staff. Consideration should be given to having one or more technologists who specialize in stent graft cases. Among the personnel involved in the case, the flow of the operation is most affected, first, by the physician team and, second, by the radiographic technologist staff.

## Company representative

A representative of the stent graft company should be present to help manage inventory, offer advice, and ensure that appropriate insertion procedures are followed. This is especially true during the initial phase of the endovascular AAA treatment program. The representative may be of assistance when problems arise.

## Operating room equipment

The primary equipment for consideration includes the radiographic imaging system, the table used for imaging, and the power injector (Figure 4.1). The location in an institution where endovascular AAA repair is performed depends on a combination of the fluoroscopic imaging capability and the sterility of the working environment. Some institutions have converted an angiographic suite into a room with operating room capabilities. This permits use of the best imaging system in the institution, but there are significant

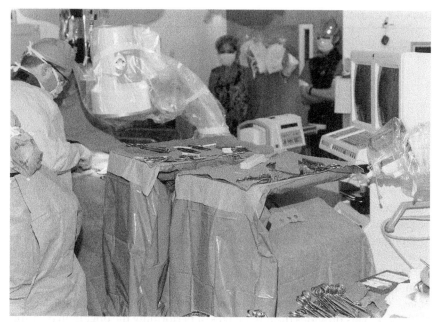

**Figure 4.1** Operating room layout. The image intensifier approaches from the patient's left, opposite the surgeon. The image monitor is also on the patient's left, in a location that is easily observed by the surgeon. The high-pressure injector is near the foot of the operating table.

barriers to creating and maintaining a sterile environment and to performing complex open operations in rooms designed for other types of procedures. In most centers, endovascular techniques have been introduced into the operating room, where sterile techniques and the concepts of graft implantation are well established. In addition, upgrading the imaging equipment, training the operating room personnel, and establishing an endovascular inventory in the vascular surgical suite provide benefits that extend to other types of vascular procedures as well.

The angiographic imaging system in the operating room may be either stationary or portable [2]. A stationary digital system with a ceiling-mounted fluoroscopic unit is desirable for its versatility, availability, and image resolution. Over the long term, most programs that are dedicated to the continuing development of endovascular techniques will require this type of "built-in" imaging unit. Unfortunately, there are several obstacles to obtaining this type of equipment. The initial cost of the equipment and room modifications, regulatory issues, and technologist staffing concerns are significant deterrents. After installation, the use of the equipment is limited to its chosen location. There are several portable digital units available that have capabilities for last-image hold, immediate playback, road mapping, and image postprocessing. Although portable fluoroscopic units are cumbersome to use and the image

**Table 4.2** Imaging requirements for endovascular repair of abdominal aortic aneurysms.

| |
|---|
| Digital imaging |
| High resolution |
| Immediate playback |
| Last-image hold and transfer |
| Road mapping |
| Postimage processing |
| Electronic storage |
| Hard copy |

quality varies, they are adequate for endovascular aneurysm repair, as has been demonstrated in many large centers. Table 4.2 lists some imaging requirements for endovascular repair of AAAs.

Options for the table include a standard operating room table with a foot extension, a dedicated but mobile radiographic table, or a fixed fluoroscopic table mounted on a single pillar. A standard operating table with a foot extension may be used by placing the patient far to one end of the table so that the image intensifier may pan over the area of interest without encountering the table base. This provides the advantages of performing the operation on a surgical table. Use of a specifically designed radiographic table, however, substantially improves image quality. Whether the radiographic table is mobile or fixed, it is usually supported on one end so that the fluoroscopic unit may pan over the patient without difficulty.

Automated pressure injection is essential for this procedure. A 20- to 25-mL bolus of viscous contrast medium must be injected over 2–3 s, usually through a 4F or 5F catheter, several times during the procedure. This requires an injection pressure of 6900–8280 kPa (1000–1200 p.s.i.). It is essential that the circulating personnel, whether nurses or technologists, have a thorough knowledge of this equipment to avoid administration of extra contrast medium and to allow the procedure to progress smoothly.

During the procedure, the surgeon is on the patient's right. The fluoroscopic unit crosses the patient from the patient's left. The television monitor may be across from the surgeon on the patient's left or near the patient's head. The injector is usually near the patient's feet and is kept in this location until after the final injection. A sterile back table located near the surgeon provides space for the guidewires, catheters, and endovascular supplies.

## Endovascular accessories and catheter inventory

General categories of supplies required for endovascular AAA stent graft placement are listed in Table 4.3. During the procedure, a rectangular back table, preferably at least 1.2 m (4 ft) long, is sterilely draped (Figure 4.2). Endovascular accessories and catheters are placed so that they are readily available. An 18-gauge, single-wall puncture needle is used for arterial access.

**Table 4.3** Supplies required for stent graft placement.

| Needles |
|---|
| Guidewires |
| Sheaths |
| Flush catheters |
| Selective catheters |
| Balloon catheters |

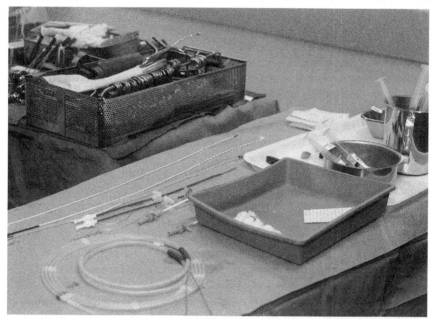

**Figure 4.2** Back table for endovascular supplies. A sterilely draped back table holds the endovascular devices that are used during stent graft placement.

The beveled tip of the needle is placed in the anterior wall of the common femoral artery. When pulsatile back bleeding is evident from the needle hub, the chosen guidewire is placed with fluoroscopic guidance.

## Guidewires

The types of guidewires that should be available are starting guidewires, steerable guidewires, and exchange guidewires. Starting guidewires (diameter, 0.035 inch; length, 145–150 cm) are made by several companies. Examples of starting guidewires are the Bentson guidewire (Cook, Inc.) and the Newton guidewire (Cook, Inc.). These guidewires are steel and have a 4- to 6-inch segment on the tip, which is soft and floppy and which is meant to pass through arterial segments without causing injury. This type of guidewire is excellent for general use and is usually the first guidewire inserted into the artery. One of these guidewires is usually placed in each femoral artery. Starting guidewires allow for initial placement of the catheter and sheath.

The second type of guidewire that should be available is the steerable, or selective, guidewire. These guidewires have an angled tip and a 1:1 turning ratio, which means that one turn of the guidewire shaft rotates the tip one turn. Because they have an angled tip, these guidewires can be used to select branch vessels and to direct catheters into specific areas. Two types of steerable guidewires are available: the Glidewire (Boston Scientific Corp., Natick, MA), which has hydrophilic coating, and the Wholey guidewire (Mallinckrodt, Inc., Hazelwood, MO), which is steel and has a tip with an adjustable curve. Steerable guidewires are used with a torque device that is fixed to the shaft of the guidewire and is used to turn and manipulate the tip of the guidewire. During stent graft placement, steerable guidewires in conjunction with selective catheters (discussed below) may be used to perform specialized tasks, including selectively catheterizing the renal artery, passing a catheter up and over the graft flow divider to the contralateral limb, and entering a graft limb. During AneuRx graft placement, a steerable guidewire is used to cannulate the contralateral gate area for insertion of the modular limb.

Steerable guidewire lengths are 150 cm, 180 cm, and 260 cm. The 260-cm length may be useful for passage through the brachial artery, through the descending aorta, and antegrade into the stent graft. The usual diameter of the steerable guidewires is 0.035 inch. However, if the flow divider of the stent graft must be crossed in an up-and-over approach, a 0.025-inch diameter guidewire is used. The 0.035-inch diameter guidewire has too much radial strength to turn the acute angle of the prosthetic graft bifurcation. The shaft of the 0.025-inch guidewire is less firm, so that the guidewire can turn this tight angle. Steerable guidewires are useful for crossing highly tortuous or stenotic arteries en route to advancing the guidewire into the abdominal aorta.

The most commonly used exchange guidewire is the stiff Amplatz guidewire (Cook, Inc.; Boston Scientific Corp.). The diameter is 0.035 inch and the length is 260 cm. The stiff shaft helps to straighten tortuous aortoiliac arteries and permits passage of the large and minimally flexible stent graft delivery devices. The firmness of the guidewire allows the operator to maintain excellent control over the treated segment until the procedure is completed. The 260-cm length is required because of the combined length of the delivery device outside the patient and the distance inside the vascular system from the femoral artery to the thoracic aorta. The leading end of the Amplatz guidewire may be placed in the thoracic aorta distal to the left subclavian artery but should not be advanced beyond that point and should be placed with the assistance of fluoroscopic guidance. After the exchange guidewire is placed, the location of the end of the guidewire outside the patient should be marked and diligently maintained throughout the procedure.

The 260-cm exchange guidewire may also be inserted through the brachial artery, passed antegrade through the aneurysmal segment, and retrieved through the femoral artery. Because the Amplatz guidewire is stiff, it should never be used as the leading edge guidewire. The most common approach is to pass a softer, more flexible or steerable guidewire into the correct location and, through a straight catheter, exchange this guidewire for the stiffer guidewire, which is used to conduct the procedure.

When an Amplatz guidewire does not provide adequate support, a Lunderquist guidewire (Cook, Inc.) may be used. The Lunderquist guidewire is stiffer than the Amplatz guidewire and is useful when a highly tortuous aorta or iliac artery creates a difficult approach to an aneurysm. Because it is stiff, the guidewire can cause endoluminal injury if not properly handled. During stent graft passage, this guidewire may be used with manual compression of the aortic aneurysm to straighten the artery temporarily.

An additional maneuver, which enhances trackability, is to place the guidewire through the left brachial artery and out the femoral artery. Whenever a stiff guidewire is in this configuration, a long sheath must be placed over it through the brachial artery to protect the origin of the left subclavian artery and the aortic arch.

## Access sheaths

Various types of sheaths may be required during stent graft placement. The initial portion of the procedure, including guidewire placement, aortoiliac arteriography, and landmarking, may be performed through 7F–9F sheaths (Pinnacle; Boston Scientific Corp.). These are standard 12- to 15-cm sheaths without any special features.

Whether placing an Ancure or an AneuRx stent graft, it is often best to place the appropriate sheath in the contralateral femoral artery. During AneuRx placement, a 16F, 35-cm sheath with a radiopaque tip (Check-Flo II introducer; Cook, Inc.) is placed through the contralateral femoral artery. The tip of the sheath may be placed in the distal aorta or proximal common iliac artery and the dilator is removed. After placement of the AneuRx stent graft body, the 16F sheath is advanced into the gate area for insertion of the contralateral limb. After the contralateral limb insertion device is placed through the sheath, the sheath is withdrawn to the hub of the insertion device so that the contralateral limb is uncovered and may be placed. After contralateral limb placement, the 16F sheath may be left in place for completion of iliac arteriography and for control of contralateral access. The Ancure contralateral limb is packaged in a specially designed delivery sheath, which allows the tip of the sheath to be locked onto the contralateral limb and used to extend the contralateral limb into the appropriate position. This device requires a short, 12F access sheath, preferably with a radiopaque marker at the tip (Cook, Inc.). If required, a larger access sheath may be used to place a diagnostic catheter through the same sheath as well.

The main body of the stent graft is introduced through the femoral artery using larger sheaths. The Ancure stent graft is passed through a flexible sheath, which is available in various lengths (Guidant Corp.). It is large enough to accommodate the Ancure delivery device and has two manually controlled hemostatic valves, a roller valve and a push valve. The AneuRx device may be inserted bareback, without the use of a sheath, or it may be placed through a 22F Keller-Timmerman sheath (Cook, Inc.) or an extra large Check-Flo introducer (Cook, Inc.). Recent modifications to the 22F sheath provide a smoother taper of the tip and a more hemostatic valve. The reasons for using a sheath are atherosclerotic disease or tortuosity of the iliac arteries approaching the aortic aneurysm, or both. The large sheaths hold a substantial volume of fluid and must be flushed regularly. A retrograde arteriogram through the side arm of the sheath requires administration of at least 15 mL of contrast medium because of the size of the sheath.

## Flush catheters

Catheters required for stent graft placement are listed in Table 4.4. Flush catheters are useful for aortography and general arteriography. These catheters have an end hole and multiple side holes to create a large blush of contrast medium on high-pressure injection. The catheter tips are rounded and atraumatic. Sometime during stent graft placement, aortoiliac arteriography is required, with use of a 5F pigtail catheter with 1-cm radiopaque markers along its length (Royal Flush II; Cook, Inc.). The catheter is placed such that the first marker is at approximately the level of the renal arteries. After aortography, the in-line length from renal arteries to bifurcation can be assessed before opening the package containing the selected stent graft for

**Table 4.4** Catheters required for stent graft placement.

Flush
    Marker pigtail[*†]
    Omni Flush[*]
Exchange
    Straight Beacon Tip[†]
Selective
    Short bent-tip: Teg-T,[†] Kumpe,[‡] Berenstain,[‡] DAV,[†] Angled Taper[§]
    Long bent-tip: MPA,[†] MPB[†]
    Hook: Rim,[†] Hook Visceral,[†] Chuang Visceral[†]
    Double curve: C1 Cobra,[†] C2 Cobra,[†] H3 Headhunter[†]

[*]AngioDynamics, Inc.
[†]Cook, Inc.
[‡] Boston Scientific Corp.
[§]Terumo Medical Corp.

placement. The Soft-Vu Omni Flush catheter (AngioDynamics, Inc., Queens-bury, NY) is another flush catheter that is quite useful in this process. After stent graft placement, the Omni Flush catheter is useful for completion aortography. During AneuRx placement, after guidewire passage through the contralateral gate, the Omni Flush may be advanced through the contralateral gate. The catheter head is rotated several revolutions inside the body of the aortic stent graft to ensure that the guidewire has appropriately entered the stent graft through the contralateral gate. The Omni Flush may also be used to direct the guidewire up and over the bifurcation of the stent graft if necessary. This catheter is available in 4F or 5F sizes and is 65 cm long. A straight 5F, 65-cm catheter with a radiopaque tip and multiple side holes (Straight Beacon Tip Royal Flush Plus; Cook, Inc.), is also useful for guidewire exchanges and for intermittent interval arteriography. This catheter is particularly useful for a magnified aortorenal arteriogram, which may be obtained immediately before placement of the stent graft distal to the renal arteries. Because the catheter is straight, it can be easily pulled back past the open proximal end of the stent graft.

## Selective catheters

Selective catheters are essential for directing guidewires during the procedure, and various shapes should be available [3]. Unlike flush catheters, selective catheters have only an end hole and no side holes. High-pressure injection is not advised. The end hole is for guidewire passage and occasional interval arteriography of side branches. The catheter heads are preshaped into configurations that may be helpful in various situations. The primary role of selective catheters in endovascular intervention is to cannulate side branches that arise from the major flow stream. For stent graft placement, these side branches also include graft limbs and other artificial components.

Selective catheters are usually used with steerable guidewires, such as the Glidewire or the Wholey guidewire. The selective catheter is used to enter an area of interest, interrogate it with arteriography, and control it by permitting passage of the guidewire, if necessary. Selective catheter placement usually begins by placing the guidewire beyond the area of interest. The selective catheter is advanced along the guidewire until its tip is within a few centimeters of the side branch or segment desired for cannulation. In some instances, the catheter tip may be advanced beyond the side branch and then withdrawn gradually to enter the orifice of the branch. This is how a cobra-shaped catheter is used to select the renal artery. In other situations, the catheter tip is placed at or just distal to the level of the branch for cannulation. The steerable guidewire is gently advanced to probe the branch while the catheter is rotated toward the branch to best direct and support the guidewire. After the steerable guidewire enters the branch, it must be advanced far enough to support the catheter as it enters the branch.

Selective catheters have a planned role in stent graft placement. When crossing an infrarenal aortic aneurysm from a femoral access, selective catheters are sometimes required to advance the guidewire, especially if the segment is tortuous or if the aneurysm is large and saccular. After placement of the AneuRx device, the contralateral gate area is cannulated using a selective catheter, often with a bent-tip or hockey-stick configuration. Occasionally, the contralateral gate cannot be approached from the contralateral femoral artery, and it must be crossed by passing a hook-shaped selective catheter up and over the graft bifurcation. The native aortic bifurcation may be crossed using an Omni Flush catheter and a steerable guidewire. Selective catheterization is occasionally required to define the location of the renal arteries or the internal iliac arteries or to treat lesions within these vessels. The C2 Cobra (Cook, Inc.) is a double-curved selective catheter that is useful for renal artery catheterization. The internal iliac artery may be entered from the contralateral side with a steerable guidewire advanced through the Omni Flush catheter used to advance across the aortic bifurcation. The internal iliac artery may be approached from the ipsilateral side using a tightly curved, hook-shaped catheter, such as the Rim catheter (Cook, Inc.) or the Rosch IMA catheter (Cook, Inc.). During Ancure device placement, selective catheterization is often required to remove the contralateral pull wire after it catches the hooks on the aortic stent. This is performed using an 8F or larger guiding catheter. Catheters with useful shapes for this include the C2 Cobra (Boston Scientific Corp.), the Renal Double Curve (Cordis Corp., Miami, FL), and the Renal Multipurpose (Pfizer, New York, NY).

Selective catheters are also commonly used to manage difficult situations that may not have been anticipated. These occasions may include, but are certainly not limited to, the following: covered side branches, misplaced graft components, kinked limbs, partially deployed devices, interrogation of endoleaks, and mistakenly withdrawn guidewires. A broad array of catheters should be available to manage both planned and unplanned maneuvers. There are scores of selective catheter shapes, and most surgeons have their favorites. Surgeons should choose a couple of selective catheters from each of the general categories: hook shaped, hockey stick, and double curved. Hook-shaped catheters may have a tighter curve, such as the Rim catheter, or a broader curve, such as the Hook or the Chuang (Cook, Inc.). Catheters with short bent-tip or hockey-stick shapes include Teg-T (Cook, Inc.), Kumpe (Boston Scientific Corp.), Berenstain (Boston Scientific Corp.), and Angled Taper Glide-Cath (Terumo Medical Corp., Somerset, NJ). The DAV catheter (Cook, Inc.) also has a short bent tip with a more acute angle for tighter corners. Catheters with longer bent tips are the MPA and MPB catheters (Cook, Inc.). Double-curved catheters include the C1 and C2 Cobra catheters (Cook, Inc.; Boston Scientific Corp.) and the H3 Headhunter (Cook, Inc.).

## Balloon catheters

During endovascular stent graft placement, balloon angioplasty is often required [4]. The Ancure device has a built-in balloon that is used to seed the hooks of the proximal and distal stents into the vessel wall. Nevertheless, additional angioplasty is often required to shape a limb of the graft or to provide additional seeding for one of the iliac hooks. Angioplasty balloons with diameters ranging from 3 to 10 mm are available on 5F shafts. Balloons with diameters ranging from 12 to 18 mm are available on 5.8F shafts. Balloons with diameters ranging from 18 to 28 mm may be mounted on shafts that are as large as 8F; these require 12F sheaths. Care must be taken to use these balloons through appropriately sized sheaths; the minimum sizes are listed on the balloon catheter packaging. Because of the open arterial access and the large size of the sheaths required for stent graft and contralateral limb placement, the placement of larger sheaths for balloon angioplasty is not as significant an issue as it is for percutaneous angioplasty. A full range of balloons should be available, from 4 to 28 mm. For balloons larger than 10 mm, compliance is greater and inflation and deflation times are increased. The pressures that the larger balloons tolerate and that are required to dilate the artery are much less than for smaller caliber balloons. Multiple companies make reliable and effective smaller balloons with diameters of 10 mm or less. The XXL series of balloons (Boston Scientific Corp.) includes diameters of 12–18 mm and the Impact series (B. Braun Medical, Inc., Bethlehem, PA) includes balloons that are 20–28 mm in diameter.

It is quite common for occlusive disease to occur in the iliac arteries, which must be treated at the time of stent graft placement. Angioplasty may be performed, either before or after the iliac limbs are in place, depending on the location and severity of disease. It may be safer to perform the balloon angioplasty through the graft limb, especially if it is juxtaposed to an aneurysmal segment of artery. If occlusive disease is severe enough that the graft cannot be placed because of a lack of access, however, the angioplasty must be performed first. Iliac disease may require angioplasty balloons that range from 7 to 12 mm in diameter. At the aortic bifurcation, or in areas where the graft limbs may impinge on each other, the "kissing-balloon" technique is most appropriate. The angioplasty catheters are managed by flushing the distal port on the balloon catheter, wiping the catheter with heparinized saline, and placing the catheter over the guidewire. The angioplasty balloon has radiopaque markers on the proximal and distal ends of each balloon for accurate placement during fluoroscopy. Often, for balloon angioplasty of the native arterial circulation, slight overdilatation of the artery is indicated to disrupt the plaque. When angioplasty is performed on the graft limb, a slight underdilatation is advised to avoid splitting the graft material.

## Conclusion

Endovascular AAA repair is facilitated significantly by careful planning for operating room equipment, personnel, and endovascular accessories. A program for insertion of aortic stent grafts requires continued development of each of these resources. As technologic advances occur, new equipment and different types of endovascular accessories may be required. The vascular specialist needs to be well informed and willing to adapt as new developments occur.

## References

1 Moore WS, Beebe HG, Chuter TAM, Fairman RM, Matsumura JS. Abdominal aortic aneurysm. In: Moore WS, Ahn SS, eds. *Endovascular Surgery*, 3rd edn. Philadelphia: WB Saunders, 2001: 421–42.
2 Diethrich EB. Endovascular suite design: an integrated approach for optimal interventional performance. In: Criado FJ, ed. *Endovascular Interventions: Basic Concepts and Techniques*. Armonk, NY: Futura, 1999: 5–16.
3 Schneider PA. More about how to get where you are going: selective catheterization. In: *Endovascular Skills: Guidewires, Catheters, Arteriography, Balloon Arthroplasty, Stents*. St Louis: Quality Medical Publishing, 1998: 63–76.
4 Schneider PA. Balloon angioplasty catheters. In: Moore WS, Ahn SS, eds. *Endovascular Surgery*, 3rd edn. Philadelphia: WB Saunders, 2001: 55–63.

# CHAPTER 5

# Essential interventional suite design, equipment, and personnel for endovascular repair of abdominal aortic aneurysms

Eric Huettl, MD, William M. Stone, MD, Richard J. Fowl, MD

## Introduction

Endovascular repair of abdominal aortic aneurysms (AAAs) has evolved into a multidisciplinary undertaking. Traditionally, vascular surgeons repaired aneurysms in the operating room and provided total care of aneurysm patients. With the emergence of endovascular grafting, however, the domain changed. Now surgeons are confronted with a new method of therapy that requires both surgical and catheter-based skills. In contrast, from the perspective of interventional radiologists, the skills required for endovascular procedures are an extension of skills long applied to stent deployment, angioplasty, embolization, and other endovascular treatments [1].

In our institution, endovascular repair of AAAs is performed in the Department of Radiology interventional angiographic suite. The decision to use the suite was multifactorial. In 1996, our institution began construction of a new hospital, which gave us the luxury of designing the interventional suite to fit our requirements, including making it operating-room compatible. We realized that endovascular repair of AAAs was heavily dependent on high-quality imaging as well as on interventional angiographic techniques and equipment. Although the traditional angiographic suite lacked several important elements, such as surgical instruments and good lighting, we agreed that these essentials could be moved more easily to the interventional suite than the imaging equipment could be moved to the operating room. We also agreed that placing a new, complete angiographic suite in an operating room would be less justifiable financially because its anticipated use would be much less than the use of similar equipment located in the Department of Radiology. Therefore, our custom-designed suite may be much more modern and better designed for endograft procedures than those available at older hospitals.

## Design of the interventional suite for endograft procedures

The most important consideration for designing the interventional suite was space. Adequate space is required for imaging, radiologic equipment, surgical equipment, radiologic and surgical personnel, and anesthetic equipment and personnel [2]. The total space in our suite includes a 532-ft$^2$ procedure room with seamless floors. However, we have found that this room is somewhat small, and at least 600 ft$^2$ would be better.

The air in the room is maintained at a positive pressure relative to the surrounding corridors. As in the operating rooms, in the procedure room there are 25 air exchanges each hour with 22% fresh air. The humidity in the procedure room, 30%, is also identical to the humidity in the operating rooms and is slightly less than at institutions in more humid climates because our institution is in a desert environment. The room temperature is maintained between 65 and 70°F (18–21°C).

The room lighting is supplemented with a ceiling-mounted surgical light and a portable floor-stand light that is routinely used during endovascular AAA repairs. A limitation of the current suite, however, is the lighting available for surgical exposure and wound closure. Ceiling-mounted, remote-controlled, high-intensity lighting is recommended for any new suite.

Anesthesiologists have brought to our attention the lack of low air returns (i.e., air-return ducts near the floor) in our suite. Low air returns are a standard at Mayo Clinic in spaces where general anesthetic gases are commonly used. There are plans to add low air returns to our angiographic suite and to include them in future procedure rooms.

Most angiographic suites have scrub facilities near the interventional room because scrub space outside the interventional suite is required for adequate sterile technique. Although angiographic procedures require sterile technique, open operative procedures require more intensive adherence to sterile technique, as does deployment of grafts. Immediately adjacent to our main angiographic suite, there is a 202-ft$^2$ case cart room that also serves as a surgical scrubbing area and inventory management area. All members of the scrub team scrub outside the interventional room before entering the room. Adequate supplies of caps, masks, and shoe covers must be available.

A major factor in the decision to perform endovascular procedures in the radiology department was the frequent need to improvise and use complex interventional skills that often require catheters, guidewires, snares, and other devices commonly used and readily available there. The endovascular team decided that it would be easier to initiate a smoothly running program by using the experience of the radiology department with this type of inventory management.

A factor in determining the amount of space required is how much anesthesia support is needed. We perform endograft placement with the patient under general anesthesia, which requires more space than the use of local anesthesia with sedation. For patient care, it seems safest to provide adequate space for the anesthetic team and their equipment in case of emergent conversion to an open procedure. Wall suction and oxygen equipment were placed in the room at the time of construction so that anesthesia could be supported fully. An anesthetic cart with all necessary equipment, including that needed for bronchoscopically guided intubation, is brought to the interventional suite before the patient enters the room. In the preoperative holding area, patients are initially evaluated and, if clinically necessary, hemodynamic monitoring lines are placed (such as arterial lines, central venous lines, Swan-Ganz catheters, and epidural catheters).

Location of the interventional suite within the hospital is important. Our suite is located near elevators to the operating room to facilitate the rapid transfer of a patient to the operating room if necessary. Convenient access to the intensive care unit is equally important. From our interventional suite, access is equally easy to both the operating room and the intensive care unit.

During the past decade, cardiac surgery has evolved to rely heavily on collaboration between heart catheterization laboratory personnel and operating room personnel. During the early years of coronary angioplasty, most hospitals required an operating room to be ready for the potentially rapid conversion from percutaneous transluminal coronary angioplasty to operative coronary artery bypass grafting. Likewise, a cardiac surgeon was required to be in the hospital before any coronary intervention. Such measures rapidly evolved, and now there are no requirements for an immediately available operating room.

Similarly, patients undergoing endografting may need potentially rapid operative intervention, but at our institution no dedicated operating room is required to be available for such an event because the chances of needing rapid conversion are small. The costs are significant for leaving an operating room empty for the rare event of needing emergent operative intervention. Although our interventional suite was designed so that urgent conversion could be performed in the suite if required, this has not occurred at our institution. When limb occlusion or complications not including hemorrhage have occurred and required operative intervention, we moved the patient to our preoperative holding area and subsequently into the first available operating room. Generally, the groin incisions are closed before the patient is transported. Even though our interventional suite is compatible with performing extra-anatomic bypasses or open aortic surgery, our preference is to perform these procedures in an operating room.

## Surgical equipment

Preparation of surgical equipment, although time consuming, is important. A sufficient supply of instruments must be available for bilateral groin incisions and dissection of the femoral arteries. Initially, we kept a full abdominal vascular setup open in the room to use for rapid conversion if needed. Data suggest, however, that complications requiring rapid conversion develop in <2% of all attempted endograft procedures [3]. With the use of balloon occlusion devices in the interventional suite, these instruments no longer need to be available. Because space is limited, we no longer keep an abdominal vascular tray open, but we do keep one near the interventional suite.

Lighting that is adequate for proper surgical exposure is absent in most angiographic suites. Lights can be mounted unobtrusively, however, so that they stay clear of all imaging equipment. Alternatively, if each surgeon wears a headlight, mounted lights are unnecessary. If headlights are used, though, there are additional space needs for the light source within the room. We have found this to be a limiting factor and have preferred to use a ceiling-mounted light.

After successful deployment of the endograft and closure of the groin wounds, the patient is awakened in the interventional suite and extubated. Recovery procedures are similar to the procedures carried out after open operative repair. For example, while the patient is transported to the postanesthetic recovery area, anesthetic personnel monitor the patient with equipment that is the same as that required for transportation from the operating room to the recovery room. The surgical team returns the instruments to the operating room to be cleaned, and the radiologic team disposes of refuse and cleans the suite in a fashion similar to how an operating room is cleaned, so that sterility can be maintained and turnover time minimized.

## Personnel

Nursing support is required from both the operating room staff and the radiologic staff. The radiologic team includes nursing support that is usually used for interventional procedures. Surgical nursing support is likewise similar to that required for open operative repair. A surgical scrub nurse or technologist, scrubbed radiologic assistant, radiologic technologist, radiologic circulating nurse, and surgical circulating nurse are required. During the procedure, all five persons are in the interventional suite; however, with cross-training only one circulating nurse needs to be present during most of the procedure.

## Imaging equipment

The decision to construct an angiographic suite in which most of the endograft procedures would be performed was based primarily on the recognition that all these procedures are extremely imaging intensive and imaging dependent. Free of any significant budgetary constraints, the team entrusted with evaluating the Department of Radiology's capital equipment purchases conducted its evaluations. This team was headed by the chair of the Vascular and Interventional Radiology Division and by the operations administrator for the Department of Radiology. After extensive evaluation of all the major vendors, the team chose a MULTISTAR Plus ceiling-mounted system (Siemens Medical Systems, Inc., Iselin, NJ). For the purposes of an imaging comparison, the team chose the Series 9600 Digital Mobile Imaging System with a Vascular Package (GE OEC, Salt Lake City, UT) as our new mobile C-arm. The capabilities and features of these two pieces of equipment show why the endovascular team decided to proceed with our program for endovascular repair of AAAs in the Department of Radiology rather than in the operating room.

The MULTISTAR Plus system is similar to other dedicated angiographic systems with its large image intensifier, digital high-quality imaging, high X-ray tube rating, digital subtraction and magnification capabilities, and high frame-rate and storage capacities. As in any dedicated angiographic system, the X-ray generator is more powerful than that of a mobile C-arm and the X-ray tube is rated higher than that of a mobile C-arm. This is important to prevent overheating of the tube during the imaging-intensive procedures and studies of the patient's abdomen. For example, the heat storage capacity of the anode in the X-ray tube in our dedicated unit is 2 million heat units as compared with 300 000 heat units for our C-arm. Another means of comparison is the anode-cooling rate, which is 405 000 heat units/min for our dedicated system and 60 000 heat units/min for the C-arm.

For AAA endovascular procedures, a large field of view is advantageous. A larger field of view allows for simultaneous imaging at the level of the renal arteries and the origin of the internal iliac arteries. Our system, like other dedicated angiographic systems, has a 16-inch image intensifier. In contrast, the standard C-arm image intensifier is 9 inches, although our vascular package C-arm has an upgraded 12-inch image intensifier. The more central aspect of the intensifier screen has better resolution, a brighter image, and less geometric distortion. Therefore, the larger the intensifier, the larger the region of optimal contrast, resolution, and minimized distortion.

Resolving power is the ability to record separate images of small objects that are placed closely together. One line pair is a line and a space. That is, the specification of 2 line pairs/mm means that there are 2 lines and 2 spaces per millimeter. Each line is 0.25 mm wide and each space is 0.25 mm wide, making each line pair 0.5 mm wide [4]. For example, the central resolution of our C-arm in the 12-inch mode is 4.4 line pairs/mm. With a smaller field and a larger magnification factor, our C-arm in the 9-inch mode resolves 4.8 line pairs/mm; in the 6-inch mode, 5.6 line pairs/mm. The superior imaging of our dedicated angiographic system allows for both a larger field of view and improved resolution. At the largest (16-inch) field of view, 4.2 line pairs/mm are resolved; in the 11-inch mode, 4.8 line pairs/mm; in the 8-inch mode, 5.6 line pairs/mm; and in the 5.5-inch mode, 6.6 line pairs/mm.

The more sophisticated image processing system of a dedicated angiographic system also contributes to imaging that is better than the best available with C-arm technology. Video monitor resolution is determined by the vertical and horizontal resolution. Vertical resolution depends on the number of vertical lines (1024 for the dedicated system and only 525 for the C-arm), whereas horizontal resolution is determined by bandwidth (>25 MHz with the dedicated system and 10.5 MHz with the C-arm). Compared with C-arm image processing, the superior image-processing system of the dedicated angiographic unit limits the amount of fluoroscopy lag. Lag, or stickiness, becomes apparent when the patient, table, or image intensifier moves during fluoroscopy and the image blurs. Another advantage of our dedicated system is the opportunity to easily add a second, slave monitor that allows for improved sight lines and better comfort for the physicians working on both sides of the procedure table.

Most dedicated angiographic systems provide better image acquisition, storage, and display than the most advanced C-arms. For example, although digital subtraction angiography with real-time subtraction and a $1024 \times 1024$ image matrix and digital real-time image filtration is standard for a dedicated system, it is not currently available with a C-arm. Higher speeds of acquisition (frame rates) are often possible with dedicated systems that have exposure rates up to 10 frames/s, while maintaining $1024 \times 1024$ image quality. More sophisticated road-mapping techniques are available with dedicated systems, although C-arms with vascular packages now feature this function in its most basic form. Dedicated systems also allow for overlay fading or for the superimposition of a real-time fluoroscopic image on a reference image of the operator's choice. Most dedicated systems also allow for an easier comparison of different angiographic scenes, including the dynamic simultaneous comparison of two series as well as options for the display of reference images beside real-time fluoroscopic images.

Dedicated angiographic systems allow for more rapid, user-friendly operation. These image processing systems, which are more automated, not only ensure optimal image quality but also enable maximal dose reduction and allow for important image-processing functions that speed and facilitate the successful completion of the procedure. For example, the capability of providing a complete overview of scenes or reference images permits the rapid and direct display of previously acquired image information. Images can be selected nonsequentially on the monitor with the use of a tableside joystick. With current C-arms, it is not possible to use quantification programs with automatic calibration during the procedure to perform such tasks as measuring distances and determining the degree of stenoses. With dedicated angiographic systems, however, these functions can be executed directly from the tableside. The image storage capacity is almost always superior with dedicated angiographic systems than with C-arms. Because endovascular procedures often require fewer stored images than other vascular and interventional radiologic procedures, the ability to rapidly and simply document images with a dedicated system is even more important. Image documentation is often a clumsy process with mobile C-arms. Also, image archiving is typically far simpler with dedicated systems that transfer images to a Digital Imaging and Communications in Medicine 3 network, such as a picture archiving and communication system, in a faster and more straightforward way than is possible with C-arms.

The speed, the almost limitless multidirectional projections, and the tableside system operation available with the sophisticated gantry system of dedicated angiographic units facilitate endovascular repair of AAAs. Unlike a manually driven and positioned C-arm, our team's ceiling-suspended gantry system features a double C-arm with adjustable isocenter angle. This feature allows for many application benefits through a wide range of angulation. The flexible positioning of the gantry, with a rotational range of 270° around the patient, allows free access to the patient from all sides. Even in the intermediate positions, which are often used to accommodate our colleagues who administer anesthesia near the head of the patient, most projections are possible. The high-speed C-arm drives at 15°/s in both left anterior oblique/right anterior oblique and cranial/caudal projections, so that it is possible to change quickly from one projection to another, which cannot be done with a mobile C-arm. In addition, gantry angle positions can be stored and recalled at the touch of a button to facilitate even more rapid selection of a particular C-arm angle. These more sophisticated gantry systems also display the image on the monitor in an automatically corrected, head-to-toe direction regardless of the gantry position. All functions necessary for an examination are integrated into the tableside control. These include motorized longitudinal movement of the gantry, C-arm, image intensifier, and table; image intensifier zoom; and collimator and filter selection and settings. With this arrangement, the physicians can accomplish all of the above tasks without giving directions to a radiologic technologist and then waiting for the actions to be carried out. Although it is a standard practice, giving directions with a mobile C-arm may result in frustrating delays and increased use of radiation.

Another important advantage that dedicated angiographic systems offer over mobile C-arms is the various measures provided to significantly decrease the radiation dose during these procedures while maintaining outstanding image quality. Foremost among these advantages is the ability to use pulsed fluoroscopy rather than continuous fluoroscopy. Although many mobile C-arms with vascular packages feature pulsed fluoroscopy, the available pulse rates of 1, 2, 4, or 8 pulses/s often generate fluoroscopic images that are unacceptable for the detailed work being performed. The pulsed fluoroscopy of a dedicated angiographic system, which can decrease the dose up to 90%, is so superior that continuous fluoroscopy is almost never used. The sophisticated electronic collimator and filter options of some dedicated systems, such as the MULTISTAR Plus, allow for additional decreases in dose. These sophisticated systems allow for radiation-free collimation by graphically displaying the position of the collimator and filters on the image monitor using the last-image hold as a guide. The physician can thereby position the collimators and filters independently without using additional real-time fluoroscopy. This may help decrease the dose by an additional 50% during fluoroscopy while improving image quality. These features do not exist with current mobile C-arms. In addition, dedicated systems measure and display the accumulated skin dose during the procedure, whereas the current C-arms provide only the fluoroscopy time, a far less useful measurement. Therefore, the ability to minimize the radiation dose to the patient and workers by using the more sophisticated radiation protection features of a dedicated angiographic system also influenced our team's choice for the location of the facilities for endovascular repairs.

## Results

During the first 2 years of using our new angiographic suite, 29 endovascular AAA and iliac aneurysm procedures were performed. Although we progressed through some of the same learning processes encountered with other new programs, none of our difficulties were attributable to performing these procedures in the interventional suite instead of in the operating room. Namely, there was one wound infection in a 280-lb patient with a large overhanging abdominal pannus, and there were no periprocedural deaths or acute surgical conversions.

## Summary

### Advantages of the interventional suite

The advantages of using the interventional suite for placing endografts include those in the following list.

1 The most important advantage is that the imaging capability in the interventional suite is vastly superior to that of the C-arm fluoroscopy that is available in the operating room. The superior image is especially helpful when cases are difficult or when intraoperative complications occur during graft deployment.

2 Multiple views of the graft are much easier to obtain in the interventional suite.

3 It is much easier to document and record the procedure on digital computer disks, and the images obtained are superior to those recorded from a C-arm fluoroscope.

4 There is less radiation exposure to both the patient and the operating team because high-quality pulsed fluoroscopy imaging is available.

5 There is much better access to various types of balloons, catheters, guidewires, and sheaths that may unexpectedly be required during the procedure, and hence there is no need for a runner between the operating room and the Department of Radiology.

### Disadvantages of the interventional suite

The disadvantages of using the interventional suite for placing endografts include those in the following list.

**1** If the duration of the endograft procedure is lengthy, the interventional suite may be occupied for hours and prevent other urgent procedures from being completed. A backup interventional room is essential for hospitals that cannot afford to have their only suite unavailable for several hours.

**2** Operating room equipment, such as an anesthesia machine and surgical instruments, must be transported to the Department of Radiology; however, this inconvenience has not caused major problems.

**3** The interventional suite is in a less sterile environment than the operating room and the potential for infection may be higher, but we have not observed this to be a significant problem.

**4** The lighting for surgical exposure and closure are inferior to the lighting in the operating room, but femoral artery exposure is a straightforward procedure and lighting has not been a major problem for the surgeons.

**5** For patients with serious comorbid conditions, the interventional suite may not be as appropriate as the operating room for management of anesthesia, but so far this has not been a problem.

## Conclusion

The ideal place for endograft placement would be a fully equipped interventional suite located in the operating room. Some hospitals are installing such equipment in one of their operating rooms, but the cost is $1–2 million. Unless the room is fully used, it is difficult to justify the expense to hospital administrators. Although we have used C-arm fluoroscopy in the operating room for endovascular procedures on a limited basis without difficulty, the Department of Radiology interventional suite has been a practical solution for providing reliable, superior imaging for endovascular repair of AAAs.

## References

1 Becker GJ, Katzen BT. The vascular center: a model for multidisciplinary delivery of vascular care for the future. *J Vasc Surg* 1996; **23**: 907–12.
2 Katzen BT, Becker GJ, Mascioli CA *et al.* Creation of a modified angiography (endovascular) suite for transluminal endograft placement and combined interventional-surgical procedures. *J Vasc Interv Radiol* 1996; **7**: 161–7.
3 Howell MH, Strickman N, Mortazavi A, Hallman CH, Krajcer Z. Preliminary results of endovascular abdominal aortic aneurysm exclusion with the AneuRx stent-graft. *J Am Coll Cardiol* 2001; **38**: 1040–6.
4 Curry TS, Dowdey JE, Murry RC Jr. *Christensen's Physics of Diagnostic Radiology*, 4th edn. Philadelphia: Lea & Febiger, 1990.

CHAPTER 6

# Diagnosis, management, and prevention of atheroembolization and contrast media–induced renal insufficiency during endovascular repair of abdominal aortic aneurysms

**Andrew Wasiluk, MD, William E. Haley, MD**

## Introduction

Patients who undergo intravascular repair of abdominal aortic aneurysms are usually elderly and frequently have diffuse erosive atherosclerosis, renal dysfunction, or other significant comorbidities. The repair procedure involves injection of contrast medium and traumatic intravascular manipulation with a catheter and stent. The risk of complications involving the kidneys may be significant.

Both cholesterol embolization (CE) and contrast media–induced nephropathy (CIN) may lead to an acute decline in renal function. Distinguishing these two entities is sometimes difficult. Although no specific treatments exist, however, establishing the correct diagnosis has important prognostic implications and may be helpful in further management. This chapter provides a review of the clinical aspects of CE and CIN.

## Cholesterol embolization

CE, also known as atheroembolic disease, was first described in 1862 by Panum [1], but it was not until 1945 that Flory [2] correlated the clinical and pathologic features and suggested that eroded atheromatous plaques in the aorta are the most likely source of embolization. Initially thought to be benign phenomena, cholesterol emboli are diagnosed frequently and are the cause of significant morbidity and mortality. They may occur spontaneously but are usually associated with anticoagulation, thrombolysis, arteriography, or vascular intervention.

Because atheromatous plaques are most common in the abdominal aorta, the visceral organs and lower extremities are commonly involved. The proximity of the kidneys and their large blood supply make them particularly susceptible to CE. There is a correlation between the severity of aortic atherosclerosis and the incidence of atherosclerotic renal disease [3,4], and renal disease may be used as a marker of visceral involvement [5].

## Incidence and risk factors

The true incidence of CE is poorly defined. Autopsy data may overestimate the incidence; clinical studies tend to underestimate it, recognizing only the most fulminant cases. The frequent delay in the onset of clinical symptoms contributes to diagnostic difficulties.

Thurlbeck & Castleman [4] found evidence of CE in 17 of 22 patients who had died within 6 months after aortic surgery.

Ramirez *et al.* [6] reviewed autopsy findings from 71 cases of patients who had died within 6 months after diagnostic angiographic procedures and found that the incidence of CE was 30% for the 20 patients who had aortograms and 25.5% for the 51 patients who had cardiac catheterization, compared with 4.3% in an age- and disease-matched population. In clinical studies, the incidence of CE after cardiac catheterization was very small [7,8].

In a review of 221 histologically proven cases of CE, Fine *et al.* [9] found evidence of aortic aneurysm in 56 patients, with 50 of these aneurysms in the abdominal aorta. At least one predisposing factor was detected for 68 patients (31%), including anticoagulation for 30 patients, vascular surgery for 20, and radiologic procedures for 39.

Thadhani *et al.* [10] reported clinical experience from one institution which involved 52 patients with histologically proven CE and consequent renal failure after invasive procedures. Twenty-three patients had abdominal aortic aneurysm. The most common invasive procedure was angiography.

## Pathogenesis and pathologic features

During procedures such as repair of abdominal aortic aneurysms, the catheter may precipitate the dislodgment of plaques, with subsequent dissemination of cholesterol emboli to the kidneys, skin, and other organs. The risk is believed to be proportional to the size and rigidity of the catheter. Anticoagulation prevents protective thrombus formation over plaques [11].

Cholesterol crystals are nondistensible and irregularly shaped, so occlusion is usually incomplete and leads to ischemic atrophy rather than infarction. Within days, an inflammatory cellular reaction occurs, resembling a reaction to a foreign body. Later, marked fibrous intimal proliferation develops. In the kidney, the arcuate and interlobular arterioles and glomerular capillaries are involved.

Lipids are dissolved by the techniques used to prepare the tissue for pathologic examination. This results in characteristic biconvex needle-shaped clefts from cholesterol crystals within the lumen of the artery (Figure 6.1). Both vascular and glomerular changes are visible, with patchy areas of renal ischemia and atrophy. Early in the acute period, cholesterol crystals may be surrounded by eosinophilic material.

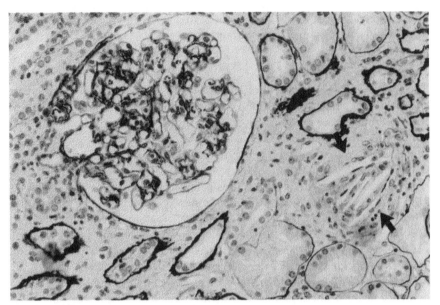

**Figure 6.1** Kidney biopsy specimen showing cholesterol crystal emboli (arrows) occluding the lumen of an arcuate artery. (Methenamine silver; original magnification ×10.) (Reprinted from Scolari F, Tardanico R, Zani R *et al.*, Cholesterol crystal embolism: a recognizable cause of renal disease, *Am J Kidney Dis* 2000; **36**: 1089–109, Copyright 2000, with permission of the National Kidney Foundation.)

## Clinical course and diagnosis

CE is a disease of the elderly, mainly affecting men with diffuse atherosclerosis. In their review of CE, Fine *et al.* [9] found concomitant coronary artery disease in 44% of the patients and hypertension in 61%. In the autopsy study by Thadhani *et al.* [10], 73% of the cases had coronary artery disease, 81% hypertension, and 69% peripheral vascular disease. The time of onset of clinical symptoms is variable; symptoms may occur within 1 day after the precipitating event or be delayed by several months. Depending on the extent of the cholesterol shower, the spectrum of the disease ranges from asymptomatic to rapidly progressive multiorgan failure. Kidneys and skin are most commonly involved.

Renal failure, which probably occurs in 50% of affected patients, may be oliguric or nonoliguric and is typically progressive, sometimes in a stepwise fashion. Partial recovery of renal function may occur, but complete recovery is exceptional. Fine *et al.* [9] found that of 129 patients with renal involvement, 40% required hemodialysis; only 20% of these regained sufficient renal function to allow discontinuation of hemodialysis.

The skin is involved in at least 35% of patients with CE; in those with skin involvement, the most common manifestations are livedo reticularis (49% of patients), gangrene (35%), cyanosis (28%), ulcerations (17%), nodules (10%), and purpura (9%) [12]. The distal pulses are usually intact.

Other organs and systems may be involved, and CE may mimic vasculitis [13,14] or pulmonary-renal syndrome [15,16], or it may cause small bowel perforation [17], acute pancreatitis, gastrointestinal tract bleeding, or stroke. Constitutional symptoms and clinical signs may be related to concomitant inflammatory changes, including fever, myalgia, and weight loss. Occasionally, accelerated hypertension is seen; it is believed to be renin-dependent.

Laboratory findings may include an increased erythrocyte sedimentation rate and eosinophilia (71–80% of patients) [18,19], a decrease in complement (39% of patients) [18], and eosinophiluria [20]. These abnormalities may be transient and hence undetected. Urinary sediment is typically nondiagnostic. Mild proteinuria frequently occurs, but only a few cases of nephrotic-range proteinuria have been reported [21].

The diagnosis of CE is frequently difficult to make on clinical grounds but should be considered for patients with acute or subacute renal failure, a history of a precipitating event such as aortic manipulation, or evidence of peripheral embolization [22,23]. Conditions to be considered for the differential diagnosis include postischemic acute tubular necrosis, radiocontrast media–induced nephropathy, acute interstitial nephritis, and systemic vasculitis. These may be distinguished in large part on the basis of the clinical course.

Biopsy findings from the affected skin or kidney should give a definite answer. Renal biopsy findings show characteristic clefts as described above, although occasionally these may be missed as a result of focal involvement. Sampling for skin biopsy should be deep because microemboli are often lodged far from any ischemic zones (Figure 6.2) [24]. In patients with visceral disease, biopsy samples of intact skin may also give positive results. In cases in which CE originates from the carotid arteries, the crystals (Hollenhorst plaques) may be seen in retinal arteries, and thus biopsy is unnecessary.

The prognosis for patients with CE is generally poor, and it often results in irreversible renal failure, amputation, and death. Overall mortality ranges from 64% to 81% [9,18]. Occasionally, renal function improves, probably as the result of management of hypertension [5], resolution of concurrent acute tubular necrosis, development of collateral flow, or hypertrophy of surviving nephrons [25].

## Management and prevention

Unfortunately, there are no specific preventive measures or therapeutic methods to be recommended for CE. Management principles include avoidance and withdrawal of anticoagulation [26], avoidance of additional intravascular procedures, treatment of hypertension, and renal replacement therapy. It has been suggested that because peritoneal dialysis does not involve anticoagulation, it may be safer than hemodialysis [27], although the overall prognosis seems to be equally poor [28].

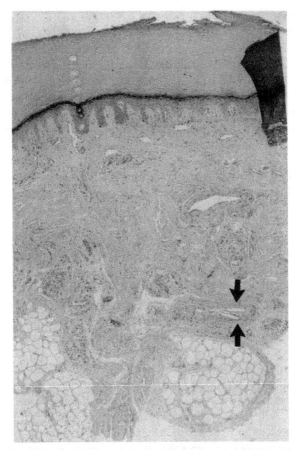

**Figure 6.2** Small artery in the derma occluded by needle-shaped clefts (arrows). (Hematoxylin-eosin; original magnification ×10.) (Reprinted from Scolari F, Tardanico R, Zani R *et al.*, Cholesterol crystal embolism: a recognizable cause of renal disease, *Am J Kidney Dis* 2000; **36**: 1089–109, Copyright 2000, with permission of the National Kidney Foundation.)

Treatment of hypertension is important. Because hypertension is renin-mediated, angiotensin-converting enzyme inhibitors and angiotensin receptor blockers should be preferred treatment agents, although in some cases renal failure has been reported to worsen after therapy with these agents was initiated [5].

Platelet inhibitors, dextran, and vasodilators have been ineffective [29]. In a few cases, statins have been described as beneficial, although the evidence is limited [30,31].

Corticosteroids have been used to treat the inflammatory response and were occasionally associated with symptomatic improvement [5,32], although they showed no benefit in most studies [6,33,34]. Some authors believe that corticosteroids may be beneficial when vasculitis-type symptoms are dominant clinically [14] or when pulmonary involvement is evident [35].

Supportive management aimed at combating three main causes of death (recurrent bouts of CE, cardiac failure, and cachexia) has improved clinical outcome [22,23].

## Contrast media–induced nephropathy

CIN is the third most common cause of hospital-acquired acute renal failure, after surgery and hypotension [36]. Although in most cases the course is benign and the renal failure is reversible, CIN may prolong the hospital stay and increase morbidity and mortality. In a retrospective study by Levy *et al.* [37], the in-hospital mortality rate was 34% for patients with CIN and 7% for patients without CIN. Various criteria have been used to define CIN in clinical studies. The most widely used criteria require a proportional increase in the concentration of serum creatinine by 25% or 50% or an absolute increase by 0.5 or 1.0 mg/dL within either 24 or 72 h. Alternative causes of increased creatinine concentrations should be ruled out. The lack of a unified definition often makes the interpretation of clinical studies of CIN difficult.

### Incidence and risk factors

Contrast agents induce a mild, transient decrease in the glomerular filtration rate in almost all patients. For significant renal failure to develop, the following additive risk factors are required:
- baseline impairment of renal function, especially in the presence of diabetes mellitus
- reduced renal perfusion (volume depletion, heart failure, cirrhosis, or nephrotic syndrome)
- concomitant use of other potentially nephrotoxic agents (e.g., aminoglycosides) or agents that may affect renal blood flow (e.g., nonsteroidal anti-inflammatory agents, angiotensin-converting enzyme inhibitors, or angiotensin receptor blockers)
- high doses or repetitive use of contrast media.

The most important risk factor for CIN is preexisting renal insufficiency. The more severe the renal failure, the more likely the development of CIN. Renal impairment prolongs elimination half-life, leading to longer exposure of the kidneys to these agents. Diabetes mellitus concomitant with renal impairment increases the risk at least twofold [38]. VanZee *et al.* [39] noted a CIN incidence of 1.4% for patients with normal renal function (creatinine <1.5 mg/dL), 9.2% for mild to moderate renal failure (creatinine 1.5–4.5 mg/dL), and 39% for severe renal failure (creatinine >4.5 mg/dL). In the subgroup with diabetes mellitus, on the basis of the same creatinine values, the incidence was 0% for patients with normal renal function, 50% for mild to moderate renal failure, and 100% for severe renal failure [39]. The risk of CIN seems to be minimal for patients with normal renal function and no other risk factors, averaging 3%

in prospective studies [40]. Diabetes mellitus per se, without renal insufficiency, does not seem to increase the risk [41]. It is important to note that older age may be considered a risk factor because it is frequently associated with decreases in renal mass, perfusion, and function. In this population, serum creatinine concentration may overestimate renal function.

The dose of contrast medium is important, although sometimes as little as 20 mL may cause renal failure in high-risk patients. In a study of patients with diabetic nephropathy and a creatinine clearance of < 30 mL/min, CIN developed in 26% of patients given < 30 mL of contrast medium, and in 79% of patients given ≥ 30 mL [42]. The acute intrarenal concentration of contrast agent is much higher after suprarenal intra-arterial injection than after intravenous administration and may possibly lead to increased toxicity.

## Pathogenesis and pathologic features

CIN may be caused by a combination of renal medullary ischemia and direct tubular epithelial cell toxicity. Injection of radiocontrast agents induces a characteristic biphasic response, with initial renal vasodilation lasting seconds to minutes which is followed by an intense and prolonged vasoconstriction that results in decreased renal blood flow [43]. Medullary ischemia is potentiated by an increase in medullary oxygen consumption resulting from increased sodium delivery to the tubules during contrast media–induced osmotic diuresis. Decreased oxygen delivery and increased oxygen consumption lead to ischemic necrosis [44]. The high energy requirements of the medulla make it particularly vulnerable to hypoxic injury.

Much research has been devoted to identification of mediators responsible for the renovascular response to radiocontrast agents. Mediators may include potent vasoconstrictors, such as endothelin or adenosine, or protective vasodilators, such as nitric oxide and prostaglandins. In experimental studies, contrast media–induced vasoconstriction was blunted by an adenosine antagonist (theophylline), endothelin receptor antagonists, prostaglandin $E_2$, prostaglandin $I_2$, and a nitric oxide precursor (arginine), whereas it was enhanced by an adenosine uptake inhibitor (dipyridamole), blockers of nitric oxide synthesis, and nonsteroidal anti-inflammatory drugs [45].

Direct toxicity leads to the generation of oxygen free radicals causing cell damage and is suggested by enzymuria after administration of contrast media and pathologic changes in the tubules. Direct toxicity might be exacerbated by hypoxia.

## Clinical course and diagnosis

CIN is usually a reversible form of acute renal failure. Typically, the serum creatinine concentration begins to increase within 24 h (in 60% of patients) or 72 h (in at least 90% of patients), peaks within 3–5 days, and returns to baseline within 7–10 days [38].

Although acute renal failure is usually nonoliguric, it may be oliguric, especially in patients with preexisting renal failure. Oliguria signifies severe injury, and affected patients tend to require dialysis [44].

In general, dialysis is necessary in 10–25% of patients with CIN, but the need is temporary in most cases [38]. Persistent renal failure may develop occasionally, usually in diabetic patients with advanced renal failure. In a study involving diabetic patients with serum creatinine levels of > 5 mg/dL, CIN occurred in 93% of the patients and was irreversible in 56% [46]. Urinanalysis is not diagnostically useful and is commonly unremarkable. Most patients, especially those who are oliguric, have low fractional excretion of sodium, which is otherwise typically seen in a prerenal state [47]. A persistent nephrogram on radiologic studies 24–48 h after the administration of contrast media has been suggested as a marker of CIN, although its clinical relevance is unknown [45].

The diagnosis of CIN is frequently obvious, based on a characteristic clinical course after the administration of contrast media. However, when an increase in creatinine concentration occurs > 72 h after contrast media administration or in low-risk patients, alternative causes should be sought. The differential diagnosis should include CE, which frequently has a more delayed onset, a more progressive course, and evidence of peripheral embolization and occasionally involves transient eosinophilia or hypocomplementemia.

## Prevention

Although numerous pharmacologic interventions have been studied and some have shown promise in animal models and limited clinical studies, none has proved effective in the prevention of CIN [45]. The intravenous administration of fluids has long been used in clinical practice to reduce the likelihood of CIN for high-risk patients, even though randomized controlled trials of its efficacy have never been conducted. Volume contraction is known to exacerbate CIN in animal experiments. The rationale for fluid administration is to correct subclinical dehydration and to counter subsequent osmotic diuresis. Half-normal saline (0.45%) has been recommended to correct volume depletion and provide water diuresis to dilute the concentration of contrast media in the urine [38].

Furosemide increases urine output and, by inhibiting active chloride transport, decreases the oxygen requirement in the medulla. Mannitol increases urine volume and expands the extracellular volume. Despite these theoretical advantages, however, the therapeutic efficacy of these agents has not been confirmed in clinical trials. In a prospective randomized study, Solomon et al. [48] found that acute renal impairment was more common in patients treated with either a combination of saline and furosemide or a combination of saline and mannitol than with saline alone (Figure 6.3).

Dopamine and theophylline have been used to prevent vasoconstriction, but not all clinical study results have been encouraging [49]. Dopamine may even increase the risk of renal injury in diabetic patients who have renal insufficiency [50]. Larger studies are needed before the routine use of such agents can be recommended. Likewise, calcium channel blockers have shown some benefit in preventing medullary vasoconstriction and preserving renal blood

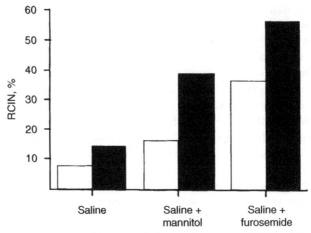

**Figure 6.3** Incidence of radiocontrast medium-induced nephropathy (RCIN) in 76 patients with renal insufficiency (serum creatinine >1.5 mg/dL) who were diabetic (black bars) or not diabetic (white bars) and who were prospectively randomly assigned to receive 0.45% saline alone for volume expansion, saline plus mannitol, or saline plus furosemide. (Reprinted from Solomon R., Contrast-medium-induced acute renal failure, *Kidney Int* 1998; **53**: 230–42, Copyright 1998, with permission of the International Society of Nephrology and Blackwell Publishing.)

flow, although there is no convincing evidence that they reduce the incidence of CIN [51].

Acetylcysteine, a free-radical scavenger, has been found to prevent the expected decline in renal function in patients with moderate renal insufficiency who also received saline hydration and a nonionic, low-osmolar contrast agent [52]. Although results of the study need confirmation in a larger number of patients, the low cost, general availability, and relative lack of toxicity have encouraged many clinicians to start using it in combination with saline hydration.

Experimental agents, such as endothelin receptor antagonists, nitric oxide precursors, prostaglandins, and atrial natriuretic peptide, have theoretical benefits, but preliminary studies are conflicting [53–55]. In a large, prospective study, low-osmolar, nonionic radiocontrast media decreased the risk of CIN in high-risk patients, but not in low-risk patients (Figure 6.4) [56]. Lack of benefit in the low-risk group may be the result of the generally low frequency of CIN.

Prophylactic hemodialysis effectively removes radiocontrast agents. Results from initial studies of this method were promising [57], but in a more recent randomized study, Lehnert *et al.* [58] found no benefit of hemodialysis in the prevention of CIN.

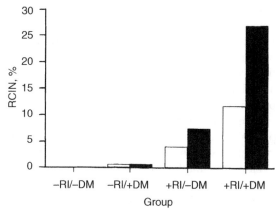

**Figure 6.4** Incidence of radiocontrast medium-induced nephropathy (RCIN) in 1196 patients who were prospectively randomly assigned to receive low-osmolar (white bars) or high-osmolar (black bars) radiocontrast media. Patients were grouped according to whether they did (+DM) or did not (−DM) have diabetes mellitus and according to whether they did (+RI) or did not (−RI) have renal insufficiency (on the basis of serum creatinine concentration ≥ 1.5 mg/dL before the procedure with contrast medium). (Reprinted from Solomon R., Contrast-medium-induced acute renal failure, *Kidney Int* 1998; **53**: 230–42, Copyright 1998, with permission of the International Society of Nephrology and Blackwell Publishing.)

## Summary of recommendations

To decrease the risk of CIN in patients undergoing endovascular repair of abdominal aortic aneurysms, the following recommendations seem reasonable.

**1** Risk for CIN should be assessed before the procedure is performed. Assessment of risk factors should include measurement of baseline concentrations of serum creatinine and estimation of volume status.

**2** Use of diuretics, angiotensin-converting enzyme inhibitors, angiotensin II receptor blockers, and nonsteroidal anti-inflammatory drugs should be discontinued 24 h before the procedure. Their use may be resumed if no significant increase in the concentration of creatinine is detected 48 h later. Patients should avoid using other potentially nephrotoxic agents, such as aminoglycosides. Patients already receiving calcium channel blockers should continue their use.

**3** For patients with renal insufficiency, acetylcysteine (600 mg, given by mouth, twice a day on the day before and on the day of the procedure) is safe and may be beneficial, pending confirmatory studies.

**4** Adequate hydration should be provided as follows:
• for outpatients with near-normal renal function, oral hydration before the procedure and infusion of 0.45% normal saline at 100 mL/h for 6 hours afterward may be sufficient [59]

- for high-risk outpatients, some authors suggest intravenous hydration for 2–4 h before the procedure with 0.5% normal saline at 100 mL/h, continued for at least 6 h after the procedure, depending on urine volume [44]
- hospitalized high-risk patients should receive intravenous hydration therapy with 0.45% normal saline at 1 mL/kg per h for 12 h before the procedure, continued for 8–12 h afterward. The protocol should be flexible, and the rate should be increased if the fluid balance becomes negative or decreased if volume overload occurs.

5 The lowest possible volume of low-osmolar and nonionic contrast medium should be used. Repetitive contrast studies should be avoided for at least 3 days. If CIN develops and another contrast procedure is absolutely necessary, it is advisable to delay it until serum creatinine concentrations decrease.

6 There is not sufficient evidence of benefit with dopamine or theophylline for these agents to be recommended for prevention of CIN; mannitol and furosemide may be detrimental. Postcontrast hemodialysis to remove the contrast agent is also not recommended.

7 The concentration of serum creatinine should be monitored at 24–48 h after the procedure. If the concentration increases above baseline, subsequent follow-up is necessary.

## References

1 Panum PL. Experimentelle Beiträge zur Lehre von der Embolie. *Virchows Arch Pathol Anat* 1862; **25**: 308–38.
2 Flory CM. Arterial occlusions produced by emboli from eroded aortic atheromatous plaques. *Am J Pathol* 1945; **21**: 549–65.
3 Sayre GP, Campbell DC. Multiple peripheral emboli in atherosclerosis of the aorta. *AMA Arch Intern Med* 1959; **103**: 799–806.
4 Thurlbeck WM, Castleman B. Atheromatous emboli to the kidneys after aortic surgery. *N Engl J Med* 1957; **257**: 442–7.
5 Dahlberg PJ, Frecentese DF, Cogbill TH. Cholesterol embolism: experience with 22 histologically proven cases. *Surgery* 1989; **105**: 737–46.
6 Ramirez G, O'Neill WM Jr, Lambert R, Bloomer HA. Cholesterol embolization: a complication of angiography. *Arch Intern Med* 1978; **138**: 1430–2.
7 Drost H, Buis B, Haan D, Hillers JA. Cholesterol embolism as a complication of left heart catheterisation: report of seven cases. *Br Heart J* 1984; **52**: 339–42.
8 Saklayen MG, Gupta S, Suryaprasad A, Azmeh W. Incidence of atheroembolic renal failure after coronary angiography: a prospective study. *Angiology* 1997; **48**: 609–13.
9 Fine MJ, Kapoor W, Falanga V. Cholesterol crystal embolization: a review of 221 cases in the English literature. *Angiology* 1987; **38**: 769–84.
10 Thadhani RI, Camargo CA Jr, Xavier RJ, Fang LS, Bazari H. Atheroembolic renal failure after invasive procedures: natural history based on 52 histologically proven cases. *Medicine (Baltimore)* 1995; **74**: 350–8.
11 Smith MC, Ghose MK, Henry AR. The clinical spectrum of renal cholesterol embolization. *Am J Med* 1981; **71**: 174–80.
12 Falanga V, Fine MJ, Kapoor WN. The cutaneous manifestations of cholesterol crystal embolization. *Arch Dermatol* 1986; **122**: 1194–8.

13  Richards AM, Eliot RS, Kanjuh VI, Blomendaal RD, Edwards JE. Cholesterol embolism: a multiple-system disease masquerading as polyarteritis nodosa. *Am J Cardiol* 1965; **15**: 696–707.

14  Rosansky SJ. Multiple cholesterol emboli syndrome. *South Med J* 1982; **75**: 677–80.

15  Case records of the Massachusetts General Hospital (Case 11–1996). *N Engl J Med* 1996; **334**: 973–9.

16  Ducloux D, Schuller V, Ranfaing E *et al.* Is atheroembolic disease a new differential diagnosis of pulmonary-renal syndrome? *Nephrol Dial Transplant* 1998; **13**: 1259–61.

17  Fujiyama A, Mori Y, Yamamoto S *et al.* Multiple spontaneous small bowel perforations due to systemic cholesterol atheromatous embolism. *Intern Med* 1999; **38**: 580–4.

18  Lye WC, Cheah JS, Sinniah R. Renal cholesterol embolic disease: case report and review of the literature. *Am J Nephrol* 1993; **13**: 489–93.

19  Kasinath BS, Corwin HL, Bidani AK *et al.* Eosinophilia in the diagnosis of atheroembolic renal disease. *Am J Nephrol* 1987; **7**: 173–7.

20  Wilson DM, Salazer TL, Farkouh ME. Eosinophiluria in atheroembolic renal disease. *Am J Med* 1991; **91**: 186–9.

21  Williams HH, Wall BM, Cooke CR. Reversible nephrotic range proteinuria and renal failure in atheroembolic renal disease. *Am J Med Sci* 1990; **299**: 58–61.

22  Belenfant X, Meyrier A, Jacquot C. Supportive treatment improves survival in multivisceral cholesterol crystal embolism. *Am J Kidney Dis* 1999; **33**: 840–50.

23  Scoble JE. Is nihilism in the treatment of atheroembolic disease at an end? *Am J Kidney Dis* 1999; **33**: 975–6.

24  Colt HG, Begg RJ, Saporito JJ, Cooper WM, Shapiro AP. Cholesterol emboli after cardiac catheterization: eight cases and a review of the literature. *Medicine (Baltimore)* 1988; **67**: 389–400.

25  Rose BD. Clinical characteristics of renal atheroemboli. Retrieved 11 August 2003, from the World Wide Web: http://www.uptodate.com.

26  Bruns FJ, Segel DP, Adler S. Control of cholesterol embolization by discontinuation of anticoagulant therapy. *Am J Med Sci* 1978; **275**: 105–8.

27  Siemons L, van den Heuvel P, Parizel G *et al.* Peritoneal dialysis in acute renal failure due to cholesterol embolization: two cases of recovery of renal function and extended survival. *Clin Nephrol* 1987; **28**: 205–8.

28  Scolari F, Bracchi M, Valzorio B *et al.* Cholesterol atheromatous embolism: an increasingly recognized cause of acute renal failure. *Nephrol Dial Transplant* 1996; **11**: 1607–12.

29  Vidt DG. Cholesterol emboli: a common cause of renal failure. *Annu Rev Med* 1997; **48**: 375–85.

30  Kawakami Y, Hirose K, Watanabe Y *et al.* Management of multiple cholesterol embolization syndrome – a case report. *Angiology* 1990; **41**: 248–52.

31  Cabili S, Hochman I, Goor Y. Reversal of gangrenous lesions in the blue toe syndrome with lovastatin – a case report. *Angiology* 1993; **44**: 821–5.

32  Boero R, Pignataro A, Rollino C, Quarello F. Do corticosteroids improve survival in acute renal failure due to cholesterol atheroembolism? *Nephrol Dial Transplant* 2000; **15**: 441.

33  Perdue GD Jr, Smith RB III. Atheromatous microemboli. *Ann Surg* 1969; **169**: 954–9.

34  Mashiah A, Pasik S, Hurwitz N. Massive atheromatous emboli to both kidneys: a fatal complication following aortic surgery. *J Cardiovasc Surg (Torino)* 1988; **29**: 60–2.

35  Vacher-Coponat H, Pache X, Dussol B, Berland Y. Pulmonary-renal syndrome responding to corticosteroids: consider cholesterol embolization. *Nephrol Dial Transplant* 1997; **12**: 1977–9.

36  Kramer BK, Kammerl M, Schweda F, Schreiber M. A primer in radiocontrast-induced nephropathy. *Nephrol Dial Transplant* 1999; **14**: 2830–4.

37 Levy EM, Viscoli CM, Horwitz RI. The effect of acute renal failure on mortality: a cohort analysis. *JAMA* 1996; **275**: 1489–94.

38 Solomon R. Contrast-medium-induced acute renal failure. *Kidney Int* 1998; **53**: 230–42. Published errata in *Kidney Int* 1998; **53**: 818; *Kidney Int* 1998; **53**: 1109.

39 VanZee BE, Hoy WE, Talley TE, Jaenike JR. Renal injury associated with intravenous pyelography in nondiabetic and diabetic patients. *Ann Intern Med* 1978; **89**: 51–4.

40 Rudnick MR, Berns JS, Cohen RM, Goldfarb S. Contrast media-associated nephrotoxicity. *Semin Nephrol* 1997; **17**: 15–26.

41 Rudnick MR, Berns JS, Cohen RM, Goldfarb S. Nephrotoxic risks of renal angiography: contrast media-associated nephrotoxicity and atheroembolism – a critical review. *Am J Kidney Dis* 1994; **24**: 713–27.

42 Manske CL, Sprafka JM, Strony JT, Wang Y. Contrast nephropathy in azotemic diabetic patients undergoing coronary angiography. *Am J Med* 1990; **89**: 615–20.

43 Murphy SW, Barrett BJ, Parfrey PS. Contrast nephropathy. *J Am Soc Nephrol* 2000; **11**: 177–82.

44 Solomon R. Radiocontrast-induced nephropathy. *Semin Nephrol* 1998; **18**: 551–7.

45 Tublin ME, Murphy ME, Tessler FN. Current concepts in contrast media-induced nephropathy. *AJR Am J Roentgenol* 1998; **171**: 933–9.

46 Harkonen S, Kjellstrand CM. Exacerbation of diabetic renal failure following intravenous pyelography. *Am J Med* 1977; **63**: 939–46.

47 Fang LS, Sirota RA, Ebert TH, Lichtenstein NS. Low fractional excretion of sodium with contrast media-induced acute renal failure. *Arch Intern Med* 1980; **140**: 531–3.

48 Solomon R, Werner C, Mann D, D'Elia J, Silva P. Effects of saline, mannitol, and furosemide to prevent acute decreases in renal function induced by radiocontrast agents. *N Engl J Med* 1994; **331**: 1416–20.

49 Abizaid AS, Clark CE, Mintz GS *et al.* Effects of dopamine and aminophylline on contrast-induced acute renal failure after coronary angioplasty in patients with preexisting renal insufficiency. *Am J Cardiol* 1999; **83**: 260–3.

50 Weisberg LS, Kurnik PB, Kurnik BR. Dopamine and renal blood flow in radiocontrast-induced nephropathy in humans. *Ren Fail* 1993; **15**: 61–8.

51 Carraro M, Mancini W, Artero M *et al.* Dose effect of nitrendipine on urinary enzymes and microproteins following non-ionic radiocontrast administration. *Nephrol Dial Transplant* 1996; **11**: 444–8.

52 Tepel M, van der Giet M, Schwarzfeld C *et al.* Prevention of radiographic-contrast-agent-induced reductions in renal function by acetylcystein. *N Engl J Med* 2000; **343**: 180–4.

53 Wang A, Holcslaw T, Bashore TM *et al.* Exacerbation of radiocontrast nephrotoxicity by endothelin receptor antagonism. *Kidney Int* 2000; **57**: 1675–80.

54 Kurnik BR, Allgren RL, Genter FC *et al.* Prospective study of atrial natriuretic peptide for the prevention of radiocontrast-induced nephropathy. *Am J Kidney Dis* 1998; **31**: 674–80.

55 Brinker JA, Sketch M, Koch JA, Bernick P. PGE 1 prophylaxis against contrast-induced nephropathy in patients with pre-existent renal compromise: results of a randomized, controlled pilot trial (abstract). *Circulation* 1998; **98**(Suppl I): I-707.

56 Rudnick MR, Goldfarb S, Wexler L *et al.*, for the Iohexol Cooperative Study. Nephrotoxicity of ionic and nonionic contrast media in 1,196 patients: a randomized trial. *Kidney Int* 1995; **47**: 254–61.

57 Moon SS, Back SE, Kurkus J, Nilsson-Ehle P. Hemodialysis for elimination of the nonionic contrast medium iohexol after angiography in patients with impaired renal function. *Nephron* 1995; **70**: 430–7.

58 Lehnert T, Keller E, Gondolf K, Schaffner T, Pavenstadt H, Schollmeyer P. Effect of haemodialysis after contrast medium administration in patients with renal insufficiency. *Nephrol Dial Transplant* 1998; **13**: 358–62.

59 Taylor AJ, Hotchkiss D, Morse RW, McCabe J. PREPARED: Preparation for Angiography in Renal Dysfunction: a randomized trial of inpatient vs outpatient hydration protocols for cardiac catheterization in mild-to-moderate renal dysfunction. *Chest* 1998; **114**: 1570–4.

# CHAPTER 7

# Anesthetic management for endovascular repair of abdominal aortic aneurysms

Monica Myers Mordecai, MD, Perry S. Bechtle, DO, Bruce J. Leone, MD

## Introduction

Anesthetic management of major vascular surgical procedures is one of the more complex areas of practice in anesthesiology. The repair of aortic aneurysms involves significant hemodynamic and metabolic stresses, particularly because the patients are usually elderly and have multiple comorbid conditions, such as ischemic heart disease, hypertension, chronic obstructive pulmonary disease, diabetes mellitus, and renal dysfunction [1].

## Treatment alternatives for abdominal aortic aneurysms

Because of the high risk of aneurysmal rupture, the current standard for the treatment of abdominal aortic aneurysms (AAAs) is open surgical repair. The procedure involves a major abdominal incision, exposure of the retroperitoneal aorta, cross-clamping of the aorta, and replacement of the aorta with a prosthetic graft. Considerable hemodynamic and metabolic stresses are associated with the surgical trauma, the increased afterload related to aortic cross-clamping, the large fluid shifts from blood loss, and the extravascular and extracellular fluid losses.

Initially, mortality for elective surgical repair of nonruptured AAAs was approximately 20%, but mortality now averages 2% in single-center studies, 4% in multicenter studies, and 7% in population-based studies [2–5]. The decrease in mortality is partly the result of improved surgical techniques and materials, more surgical experience, and improvements in anesthetic management, monitoring, and postoperative care [3]. Although mortality has decreased, aortic surgery is still associated with significant morbidity and the potential for a long convalescence. Morbidity related to open surgical repair may result from myocardial infarction, renal failure, pulmonary dysfunction, hepatic failure, ischemic bowel, spinal cord ischemia, embolism, or stroke. Furthermore, some patients may not be eligible for the operation because the risks are considered too high. These factors have led to the investigation of alternative methods for management of AAAs.

Endovascular aneurysm repair (EVAR) is less invasive than open surgical repair and is used for various aortic diseases, most commonly AAAs. The clinical use of this technique was first described by Parodi *et al.* [6] in 1991.

The selection of aneurysms suitable for EVAR is based on several factors, including the morphologic features and location of the aneurysm. The ideal candidate is an infrarenal aneurysm with appropriate proximal and distal attachment sites [7].

The procedure is usually performed in an operating room with interventional capabilities. The patient is prepared and draped for standard surgical repair in case conversion to an open surgical procedure is necessary. Access is typically infrainguinal, through femoral artery exposure. Large-diameter sheaths are placed into the aorta by means of a femoral arteriotomy. The delivery system for the stent graft is inserted through a retractable sheath. Intravenous contrast medium is used throughout the procedure to define aortic branches and to confirm proper placement and function of the graft.

## Advantages of endovascular aneurysm repair

Initial studies have found that, when compared with conventional open surgical repair, EVAR has considerable advantages, including less blood loss, less use of an intensive care unit, shorter duration of hospitalization, and faster recovery [8]. With EVAR, the approach is infrainguinal, which avoids the need for a major abdominal incision and exposure of the retroperitoneal aorta. Interruptions of aortic blood flow are shorter than in open surgical repair, and aortic cross-clamping is avoided.

During conventional surgical repair, the placement of an aortic cross-clamp causes an immediate increase in afterload and systemic vascular resistance, and the heart compensates for the increased myocardial oxygen demand with an increase in coronary blood flow [9]. Patients with limited cardiac reserve thus may not tolerate the hemodynamic consequences of aortic cross-clamping. Cardiovascular complications observed in patients undergoing elective AAA repair almost always occur at the time of infrarenal aortic cross-clamping [10]. Metabolic disturbances due to aortic cross-clamping include metabolic acidosis and release of multiple mediators associated with the stress response [9].

For the repair of AAAs, EVAR has been shown to cause significantly less intraoperative hemodynamic and metabolic stress than conventional open surgery [11]. Plasma catecholamine concentrations and changes in cardiovascular variables and acid-base status were all greater with open surgical repair than with EVAR [12]. The decreased stress response with EVAR may also be attributed to decreased bowel ischemia, endotoxemia, and cytokine generation [13]. Each technique produces a different biologic response: EVAR induces an inflammatory response, whereas conventional open repair induces responses associated with extensive surgical trauma and reperfusion injury [14].

Other advantages of EVAR include improved postoperative respiratory function and analgesic control [15]. Complications in patients treated with EVAR tend to be localized vascular complications that may be corrected at the time of surgery and are less severe than the remote systemic complications predominating in patients treated with open repair [8].

Because EVAR is a localized procedure, another advantage is the possible use of regional and intravenous analgesia or local anesthesia administered as a paravertebral blockade as an alternative to general anesthesia.

## Management of patients undergoing endovascular aneurysm repair

### Preoperative evaluation

As with open repair, considerations for anesthetic management of patients undergoing EVAR begin with a thorough preoperative evaluation to determine comorbidity affecting cardiac, pulmonary, renal, or cerebral function; to allow optimization of medical therapies; and to assess risk factors known to increase perioperative morbidity and mortality.

Because myocardial infarction is by far the most common cause of morbidity and mortality in the surgical repair of AAAs, initial evaluation begins with the heart. Preexisting cardiac disease is the most significant factor affecting immediate survival. The prevalence of coronary artery disease in patients presenting for vascular surgery is high [16]. Hertzer *et al.* [17] found that only 8% of patients had normal coronary arteries and 31% had severe coronary artery disease. Additional cardiac testing, such as Holter monitoring, stress testing, echocardiography, or cardiac catheterization, can assist in stratifying cardiac risk. The mortality rate is increased threefold if patients have a history of congestive heart failure, an ejection fraction <30%, myocardial infarction within the past 6 months, or angina [18].

Katz *et al.* [4] found significantly increased operative mortality rates among patients with ischemic heart disease who had operations performed before 1984. A decrease in mortality observed since 1984 may be partly attributed to better detection of cardiac disease in this patient population and to improvements in anesthetic management and monitoring. Performance of coronary angiography allows surgical therapy for coronary artery disease, thus decreasing early mortality after elective surgical procedures for repair of AAAs [19]. If coronary artery disease, congestive heart failure, or uncontrolled hypertension is detected, medical therapy can be optimized and the necessity for more invasive intraoperative monitoring, with techniques such as pulmonary artery catheterization or transesophageal echocardiography, can be determined.

Chronic obstructive pulmonary disease is a risk factor for patients with AAAs. For patients with known or suspected pulmonary disease, preoperative testing should include chest radiography, arterial blood gas analysis, and bedside spirometry. Pulmonary function testing is used to predict postoperative pulmonary complications and the need for postoperative ventilation, to evaluate the response to bronchodilator therapy, and to define the nature of the disease (obstructive, restrictive, or mixed disease). An increased risk of postoperative pulmonary dysfunction is indicated by pulmonary disease, as demonstrated by a partial pressure of arterial oxygen of <60 mmHg on room air; hypercarbia; forced expiratory volume in 1 s of <2 L; or a vital capacity <50% of that predicted [20]. Postoperative pulmonary function is also affected by the site of the operation; for example, abdominal surgery decreases vital capacity and the ability to cough.

The correlation between chronic obstructive pulmonary disease and AAAs may be related to a history of significant tobacco abuse among patients with chronic obstructive pulmonary disease. The benefits of discontinuing smoking before the operation are not clear. Immediately after discontinuation, carboxyhemoglobin levels decrease and oxygen availability increases. The return of mucociliary function takes weeks, however, and it is unclear whether postoperative pulmonary dysfunction is lessened.

Preexisting renal failure has been associated with a mortality rate as high as 41% in conventional repair of AAAs [4]. Preoperative laboratory testing should include determination of concentrations of serum electrolytes, serum urea nitrogen, and creatinine in addition to urinalysis. Intraoperatively, renal function can be compromised by vascular interruption or by angiographic contrast media–induced acute tubular necrosis. Maintenance of intravascular volume and urine output may decrease the risk of postoperative renal failure, which is the second most common cause of death. Additional risk factors associated with in-hospital death include female sex and advanced age [4].

Because atherosclerosis may affect cerebral vessels, the physical examination should include auscultation of the carotid arteries for the presence of bruits. The baseline range of blood pressure for the patient should be determined. Intraoperative hypotension requested during placement of the endoluminal prosthesis may compromise cerebral blood flow in patients with cerebrovascular disease.

In addition to collecting the patient history and performing a physical examination, preoperative measures include explaining the intraoperative events to the patient to decrease anxiety and premedicating the patient with a low dose of benzodiazepine.

## Monitoring

The goals of intraoperative management are to provide hemodynamic stability while preserving cardiac and renal blood flow and maintaining intravascular volume, adequate oxygenation, and body temperature. Because of the high prevalence of coronary artery disease in patients undergoing aortic surgery, a continuous monitor for ischemia is required. The most sensitive and least invasive method of monitoring for myocardial ischemia is to follow electrocardiographic leads II and $V_5$ for continuous ST-segment trend analysis, which can detect up to 95% of the intraoperative ischemic events. More invasive means of monitoring ischemia include posteroanterior catheter analysis of waveforms, pressure trends of cardiac output, and two-dimensional transesophageal echocardiographic detection of regional wall motion abnormalities.

An arterial line is required for continuous blood pressure monitoring and can also be used for sampling arterial blood gases, hematocrit, and activated clotting time as needed. Because of the systemic nature of atherosclerosis, before placement of a radial arterial line, blood pressure should be checked in both arms to detect any differences. Central venous access is recommended to determine and maintain intravascular volume and to provide central delivery of vasopressors. In patients with poor left ventricular function or renal failure, use of a pulmonary artery catheter or transesophageal echocardiography may provide a more accurate assessment of intravascular volume and cardiac function. A Foley catheter is used for an additional measure of volume status. Urine output reflects maintenance of renal blood flow. Because patients are surgically prepared and draped for a full open procedure, which leaves a large area of skin exposed, body temperature should be followed closely and maintained appropriately. Additionally, the left antecubital fossa may be surgically prepared to be available for arterial access during the procedure.

## Intraoperative concerns

Because of the technical aspects of the stent graft system and procedure, EVAR of an aortic aneurysm presents unique challenges for the intraoperative management and development of a safe anesthetic plan. EVAR is less invasive than open surgical repair and less likely to induce hemodynamic stress, yet it has many of the same risks and complications of conventional aortic surgery, such as injury to the iliac artery by the introducer apparatus or massive, sudden blood loss owing to aortic leak or rupture. Sudden blood loss is devastating, with a mortality rate that exceeds 50%.

After the patient is brought to the operative suite, the appropriate lines for hemodynamic monitoring should be placed, in addition to large-bore intravenous access. The patient is surgically prepared and draped for a full open procedure. When local anesthesia is used, patient position is a concern because movement can make correct radiographic positioning of the graft difficult.

Intraoperative fluids must be managed closely, with early replacement of preoperative fluid deficits and maintenance of intravascular volume. After the baseline activated clotting time is determined, anticoagulation is begun with an initial heparin dose of 5000 units administered intravenously before insertion of the arterial catheters. Significant blood loss may occur during placement of the introducer sheaths and during manipulation of the stent graft system, but hemostatic valves have greatly decreased blood loss during stent manipulation.

Balloon expansion during placement of the stent causes short periods of aortic occlusion, which typically last 30–60 s and are usually not hemodynamically significant. Bradycardia and hypotension are occasionally associated with this arterial manipulation. During deployment of balloon-expandable devices, hypotension may be used to decrease the proximal pulse pressure of systole to ensure proper placement of the stent by avoiding the necessity of applying force on the stent distally. Especially with thoraco-abdominal grafts, migration is more pronounced when the graft is placed more proximally to the heart. Hypotension may also decrease the risk of aortic dissection or rupture and of myocardial stress from the increased afterload during placement.

Agents used to induce hypotension during this period include nitroglycerin (most commonly) and sodium nitroprusside; maneuvers include induced ventricular fibrillation, adenosine-induced asystole, and the Valsalva maneuver [21,22]. The time during deployment of the stent graft system is a critical intraoperative period. The differential diagnosis for acute hypotension after stent deployment includes acute aortic rupture, cardiac failure due to increased afterload of aortic occlusion, macroembolization of thrombotic material, local anesthetic toxicity, allergic reaction to a medication or contrast medium, and side effects of the maneuvers to induce hypotension.

Intraluminal manipulation with guidewires or the stent graft system has been related to various intraoperative complications. Macroembolization or microembolization can be devastating. A fatal cerebral embolism manifesting intraoperatively as sudden respiratory arrest has been reported [23]. Intra-cardiac wire misplacement can cause acute aortic insufficiency and hypotension [24]. Additional complications reported with EVAR include endoleak (persistent communication between the aneurysm and the aortic circulation after graft placement); malposition or migration of the graft which compromises renal, abdominal, pelvic, or lower extremity blood flow; and aneurysmal rupture. Conversion to open surgery in itself may be associated with increased mortality [25].

The practice of anesthesia has expanded from the operating room to other areas of the hospital, and EVAR is performed in interventional radiologic suites at some institutions. When used for this procedure, such suites must have full surgical capabilities for open surgical repair of AAAs or have an operating room immediately available in the event of rupture or conversion to open repair procedures. The possibility must be considered that a patient with an acutely ruptured aneurysm, iliac artery, or proximal aorta would have to be transported while attempts are made to rapidly infuse fluid, provide inotropic support, and monitor the patient. Urgent conversion to open repair procedures has a mortality rate >40% [26].

## Postoperative care

Postoperative recovery after EVAR does not usually require the use of an intensive care unit. The patients are typically ambulatory and eat a regular diet on the first postoperative day. Analgesic requirements are minimal and can be managed with nonsteroidal anti-inflammatory medications or small boluses of narcotics. Postimplantation syndrome owing to a systemic inflammatory response to the graft material may occur postoperatively, with fever, leukocytosis, and increased C-reactive protein concentrations [27,28]. Hyperpyrexia associated with tachycardia warrants continued monitoring of hemodynamics among patients with cardiac disease. With an uncomplicated perioperative course, the length of hospital stay is typically 48 h.

## Anesthetic techniques

As reported in 1991 by Parodi *et al.* [6], the first placements of intraluminal grafts were performed under local or limited epidural anesthesia. For the experimental procedure, these investigators selected five high-risk patients with serious comorbidities, such as severe chronic obstructive pulmonary disease, acute stroke, severe asthma, or ejection fraction <20%. Parodi *et al.* [6] determined that the transfemoral approach allowed for the procedure to be performed under local or limited epidural anesthesia without the morbidity of a high regional block or an inhalational general anesthetic. Various anesthetic techniques for the management of endovascular surgery have since been reported. These include general anesthesia, combined general and regional anesthesia, epidural anesthesia, and combined spinal–epidural anesthesia, as well as local anesthesia with sedation.

Most groups initially performed EVAR with general anesthesia. For both the surgeons and the anesthesiologists, this choice was probably related to the uncertainties of performing a new surgical technique. For example, according to a report of clinical experience at one institution, EVAR procedures were performed with general anesthesia until acceptable operating room times and a low risk of surgical complications were determined; after the first seven operations, most were done with local anesthesia [29].

A safe anesthetic can be administered by a vigilant and capable anesthesiologist using any of the techniques mentioned above. The question is whether any particular anesthetic technique is superior for achieving the goals of anesthetic management, i.e., providing hemodynamic stability with minimal use of inotropic agents, maintaining intravascular volume without excessive fluid administration, and preserving cardiac, pulmonary, renal, and cerebral blood function.

### General anesthesia

For the induction and maintenance of general anesthesia, the choice of medications and means of hemodynamic monitoring are based on the patient's cardiac function. Patients with preserved left ventricular function generally tolerate the depressant effects of intravenous and inhaled anesthetic agents with appropriate compensatory mechanisms. General anesthesia typically consists of a balanced technique with a low-dose inhalational agent, narcotics, and muscle relaxants. For patients with compromised left ventricular function, a narcotic-based technique provides greater hemodynamic stability.

General anesthesia provides airway control throughout the procedure, allows for stable hemodynamic management, accommodates variations in the duration of the operation, eliminates the possibility of patient movement, and allows for the control of respiratory movement during fluoroscopy. Furthermore, the patient is asleep for additional line placement and can tolerate lying supine on the operating table during long operations. In a few nonrandomized retrospective studies of anesthetic technique, general anesthesia was associated with more hypotensive episodes, increased fluid requirements, and an increased use of inotropic support than regional or local anesthesia [29–35].

## Regional anesthesia

### Types of regional anesthesia

Spinal, epidural, and combined spinal–epidural techniques have been used for EVAR. The sensory level of anesthetic blockade needed for this surgery extends from the T8 through the T10 dermatomes. This provides anesthesia for the infrainguinal surgical field and for peritoneal retraction, if needed for iliac artery exposure. The block can be performed in the low lumbar region. Published descriptions of regional techniques and local anesthetic agents for EVAR include epidural catheter dosing with bupivacaine (0.5%) to achieve an adequate sensory level and spinal anesthesia with bupivacaine. The level of sensory anesthesia required for EVAR has fewer hemodynamic side effects than the high thoracic level needed for open surgical repair.

The advantages of epidural anesthesia over other regional techniques include the ability to slowly titrate the local anesthetic to achieve anesthesia at the appropriate level of sensory dermatomes and to accommodate variations in the duration of the procedure. Also, slow titration of an epidural anesthetic allows for compensatory mechanisms to minimize hemodynamic changes.

Spinal anesthesia is more difficult to titrate slowly to a specific level and is inadequate if the operation is prolonged unexpectedly. The use of combined spinal and epidural techniques has increased fluid requirements by up to 2 L [34].

### Advantages of regional anesthesia

At some institutions the choice of anesthetic is based on surgical approach, with regional anesthesia used for the iliac approach and local anesthesia for the femoral approach [29]. Regional anesthesia has a proven advantage over general anesthesia for postoperative pulmonary function. General anesthesia with mechanical ventilation can cause decreased lung volume, ventilation–perfusion mismatch, decreased functional residual capacity, atelectasis, impaired ciliary function with thickened secretions predisposing to postoperative pulmonary dysfunction, and infections. Whether regional anesthesia is beneficial for patients with compromised myocardial function is controversial because of the difficulty in demonstrating differences in morbidity and mortality.

In attempting to identify differences in outcome, many studies have compared general anesthesia with combined general–epidural anesthesia for surgical procedures that have significantly more surgical trauma or that require a higher thoracic level of anesthesia than required for EVAR. The hemodynamic effects owing to increased venous capacitance and decreased preload of a low lumbar epidural anesthetic titrated slowly are minimal. If blood pressure is maintained, myocardial function should not be significantly affected. Regional anesthesia for EVAR has been reported for a series of 21 patients with no periods of clinically significant hypotension during the procedure [33]. The use of vasopressors and the median fluid balance are lower with the use of regional anesthesia than with general anesthesia for EVAR [29].

Other benefits of regional anesthesia over general anesthesia include a shorter hospital stay after the operation [32]. For certain procedures, intraoperative blood loss has been reported to be less with regional anesthesia than with general anesthesia. For EVAR specifically, intraoperative blood loss seems to be similar between regional anesthesia and general anesthesia [28,29,32]. Because such low levels of anesthesia are required for EVAR, the procedure is not accompanied by the theoretical disadvantages of regional anesthesia, such as difficulty controlling hemodynamics in a bleeding patient who has a high sympathectomy or postoperative fluid overload when the block recedes. The incidence of thrombotic events in peripheral grafts, coronary arteries, and lower extremity veins is lower with regional anesthesia than with general anesthesia. This is probably because the hypercoagulable state is attenuated in patients undergoing peripheral vascular procedures, which may provide potential benefits.

Potential disadvantages of regional anesthesia include difficulties in keeping the patient comfortable while lines are being placed and while the supine position must be maintained on the operating table, when fluoroscopic imaging without patient movement is vital.

### Risk of epidural hematoma
Patients undergoing peripheral vascular surgery while receiving intraoperative heparinization can have regional anesthesia administered safely, with a low risk of spinal or epidural hematoma. Theoretical concerns about placement of a catheter in a patient who will receive anticoagulation intraoperatively should not restrict the use of regional anesthesia if results of coagulation tests are normal when the block or epidural catheter is placed and before it is removed. Neurologic function should be monitored postoperatively.

### Local anesthesia
For the transfemoral approach, local anesthesia is well tolerated and provides greater hemodynamic stability than other anesthetic techniques, as demonstrated by the decreased use of inotropic agents [36,37]. Intravenous sedation regimens include titration of benzodiazepines with or without continuous

**Table 7.1** Comparison of general, epidural, and local anesthesia for endovascular aneurysm repair.*

| Anesthesia | No. of patients | Fluid administration, mL | Vasopressor use, % of patients | Operating time, min |
|---|---|---|---|---|
| Local | 63 | 1000 ± 147 | 8 | 100 |
| Epidural | 8 | 1460 ± 446 | 25 | 125 |
| General | 20 | 1950 ± 590 | 50 | 172 |

*Data from Bettex *et al.* [29].

infusions of propofol or narcotics. Modifications in surgical technique and catheter technology have simplified parts of the procedure, e.g., by decreasing clamping time, leg ischemia, and pain for patients. Henretta *et al.* [35] first demonstrated the feasibility of local anesthesia with intravenous sedation as a safe alternative in 47 patients. Their series had 48 consecutive patients, but one patient was excluded because of severe esophageal stricture. In one patient, the local anesthetic technique was converted to a general anesthetic technique because a retroperitoneal approach was needed for iliac artery repair. Only one patient was admitted to the intensive care unit. In a retrospective analysis of 91 patients, local anesthesia was superior to both general and epidural anesthesia on the basis of decreased fluid requirements, decreased operating time, and decreased use of vasopressors (Table 7.1) [29].

As for any surgical procedure with local or regional anesthesia, preparations must be made for switching to general anesthesia if conversion to open surgical techniques becomes necessary or if further access to the iliac arteries is needed.

## Summary

Indications for EVAR extend well beyond elective repair of AAAs. EVAR procedures have been used to repair ruptured abdominal aneurysms in patients with contained retroperitoneal bleeding, thoracoabdominal aneurysms, and aortic injuries caused by blunt trauma. Many of these operations are performed under local anesthesia. As larger series of clinical experiences are described from an anesthetic perspective and randomized prospective trials are performed, the validity of results of earlier studies comparing anesthetic techniques can be reevaluated. Modifications of endografts include one system of percutaneous transfemoral prosthesis deployment [38]. As the technology in this rapidly evolving surgical field continues to develop, it is likely that most of the procedures will be performed with the administration of local anesthesia. Even when surgical and anesthetic techniques are less invasive, patients have a high incidence of severe coexisting diseases and continue to require complex management throughout the perioperative period.

# References

1 Ross R. The pathogenesis of atherosclerosis: an update. *N Engl J Med* 1986; **314**: 488–500.
2 Ernst CB. Abdominal aortic aneurysm. *N Engl J Med* 1993; **328**: 1167–72.
3 Crawford ES, Saleh SA, Babb JW III *et al.* Infrarenal abdominal aortic aneurysm: factors influencing survival after operation performed over a 25-year period. *Ann Surg* 1981; **193**: 699–709.
4 Katz DJ, Stanley JC, Zelenock GB. Operative mortality rates for intact and ruptured abdominal aortic aneurysms in Michigan: an eleven-year statewide experience. *J Vasc Surg* 1994; **19**: 804–15.
5 Zarins CK, White RA, Schwarten D *et al.* AneuRx stent graft versus open surgical repair of abdominal aortic aneurysms: multicenter prospective clinical trial. *J Vasc Surg* 1999; **29**: 292–305.
6 Parodi JC, Palmaz JC, Barone HD. Transfemoral intraluminal graft implantation for abdominal aortic aneurysms. *Ann Vasc Surg* 1991; **5**: 491–9.
7 May J, White GH, Yu W *et al.* Results of endoluminal grafting of abdominal aortic aneurysms are dependent on aneurysm morphology. *Ann Vasc Surg* 1996; **10**: 254–61.
8 Brewster DC, Geller SC, Kaufman JA *et al.* Initial experience with endovascular aneurysm repair: comparison of early results with outcome of conventional open repair. *J Vasc Surg* 1998; **27**: 992–1003.
9 Gelman S. The pathophysiology of aortic cross-clamping and unclamping. *Anesthesiology* 1995; **82**: 1026–60.
10 Dunn E, Prager RL, Fry W, Kirsh MM. The effect of abdominal aortic cross-clamping on myocardial function. *J Surg Res* 1977; **22**: 463–8.
11 Baxendale BR, Baker DM, Hutchinson A *et al.* Haemodynamic and metabolic response to endovascular repair of infra-renal aortic aneurysms. *Br J Anaesth* 1996; **77**: 581–5.
12 Thompson JP, Boyle JR, Thompson MM *et al.* Cardiovascular and catecholamine responses during endovascular and conventional abdominal aortic aneurysm repair. *Eur J Vasc Endovasc Surg* 1999; **17**: 326–33.
13 Elmarasy NM, Soong CV, Walker SR *et al.* Sigmoid ischemia and the inflammatory response following endovascular abdominal aortic aneurysm repair. *J Endovasc Ther* 2000; **7**: 21–30.
14 Swartbol P, Norgren L, Albrechtsson U *et al.* Biological responses differ considerably between endovascular and conventional aortic aneurysm surgery. *Eur J Vasc Endovasc Surg* 1996; **12**: 18–25.
15 Boyle JR, Thompson JP, Thompson MM *et al.* Improved respiratory function and analgesia control after endovascular AAA repair. *J Endovasc Surg* 1997; **4**: 62–5.
16 Hertzer NR, Young JR, Kramer JR *et al.* Routine coronary angiography prior to elective aortic reconstruction: results of selective myocardial revascularization in patients with peripheral vascular disease. *Arch Surg* 1979; **114**: 1336–44.
17 Hertzer NR, Beven EG, Young JR *et al.* Coronary artery disease in peripheral vascular patients: a classification of 1000 coronary angiograms and results of surgical management. *Ann Surg* 1984; **199**: 223–33.
18 Brown OW, Hollier LH, Pairolero PC, Kazmier FJ, McCready RA. Abdominal aortic aneurysm and coronary artery disease. *Arch Surg* 1981; **116**: 1484–8.
19 Busch T, Sirbu H, Aleksic I, Friedrich M, Dalichau H. Importance of cardiovascular interventions before surgery for abdominal aortic aneurysms. *Cardiovasc Surg* 2000; **8**: 18–21.
20 Tisi GM. Preoperative identification and evaluation of the patient with lung disease. *Med Clin North Am* 1987; **71**: 399–412.

21 Nishikimi N, Usui A, Ishiguchi T *et al.* Vena cava occlusion with balloon to control blood pressure during deployment of transluminally placed endovascular graft. *Am J Surg* 1998; **176**: 233–4.

22 Kahn RA, Marin ML, Hollier L, Parsons R, Griepp R. Induction of ventricular fibrillation to facilitate endovascular stent graft repair of thoracic aortic aneurysms. *Anesthesiology* 1998; **88**: 534–6.

23 Zaugg M, Lachat ML, Pfammatter T, Cathomas G, Schmid ER. Sudden respiratory arrest resulting from brainstem embolism in a patient undergoing endovascular abdominal aortic aneurysm repair. *Anesth Analg* 2001; **92**: 335–7.

24 Sutton DC, Rother A. Endoluminal abdominal aortic aneurysm repair complicated by intracardiac guidewire placement and massive transfusion. *Anesth Analg* 2000; **91**: 89–91.

25 May J, White GH, Yu W *et al.* Conversion from endoluminal to open repair of abdominal aortic aneurysms: a hazardous procedure. *Eur J Vasc Endovasc Surg* 1997; **14**: 4–11.

26 May J, White GH, Waugh R *et al.* Adverse events after endoluminal repair of abdominal aortic aneurysms: a comparison during two successive periods of time. *J Vasc Surg* 1999; **29**: 32–7.

27 Blum U, Voshage G, Lammer J *et al.* Endoluminal stent-graft for infrarenal abdominal aortic aneurysms. *N Engl J Med* 1997; **336**: 13–20.

28 Eberle B, Weiler N, Duber C *et al.* Anesthesia in endovascular treatment of aortic aneurysm: results and perioperative risks. *Anaesthesist* 1996; **45**: 931–40 [in German].

29 Bettex DA, Lachat M, Pfammatter T *et al.* To compare general, epidural and local anaesthesia for endovascular aneurysm repair (EVAR). *Eur J Vasc Endovasc Surg* 2001; **21**: 179–84.

30 Greiff JM, Thompson MM, Langham BT. Anaesthetic implications of aortic stent surgery. *Br J Anaesth* 1995; **75**: 779–81.

31 Baker AB, Lloyd G, Fraser TA, Bookallil MJ, Yezerski SD. Retrospective review of 100 cases of endoluminal aortic stent-graft surgery from an anaesthetic perspective. *Anaesth Intensive Care* 1997; **25**: 378–84.

32 Cao P, Zannetti S, Parlani G *et al.* Epidural anesthesia reduces length of hospitalization after endoluminal abdominal aortic aneurysm repair. *J Vasc Surg* 1999; **30**: 651–7.

33 Aadahl P, Lundbom J, Hatlinghus S, Myhre HO. Regional anesthesia for endovascular treatment of abdominal aortic aneurysms. *J Endovasc Surg* 1997; **4**: 56–61.

34 Yeager MP, Fillinger MP, Lundberg J. Cardiothoracic and vascular surgery. In: Brown DL, ed. *Regional Anesthesia and Analgesia*. Philadelphia: WB Saunders, 1996: 512–36.

35 Henretta JP, Hodgson KJ, Mattos MA *et al.* Feasibility of endovascular repair of abdominal aortic aneurysms with local anesthesia with intravenous sedation. *J Vasc Surg* 1999; **29**: 793–8.

36 Lachat M, Pfammatter T, Turina M. Transfemoral endografting of thoracic aortic aneurysm under local anesthesia: a simple, safe and fast track procedure. *Vasa* 1999; **28**: 204–6.

37 Lachat M, Pfammatter T, Bernard E *et al.* Successful endovascular repair of a leaking abdominal aortic aneurysm under local anesthesia. *Swiss Surg* 2001; **7**: 86–9.

38 Papazoglou K, Christu K, Iordanides T *et al.* Endovascular abdominal aortic aneurysm repair with percutaneous transfemoral prostheses deployment under local anaesthesia: initial experience with a new, simple-to-use tubular and bifurcated device in the first 27 cases. *Eur J Vasc Endovasc Surg* 1999; **17**: 202–7.

# PART II

---

# Commercially available stent graft systems

# CHAPTER 8

# Commercially available endovascular stent grafts

Timothy A. Hipp, MD, Albert G. Hakaim, MD

## Introduction

The first report of endovascular aneurysm repair (EVAR), in the English-language literature, was that of Parodi *et al.* [1] in 1991. Since that time, various stent graft devices have been developed. Thus far, five devices have received US Food and Drug Administration (FDA) approval: Ancure (Guidant Corp., Menlo Park, CA), AneuRx (Medtronic, Inc., Minneapolis, MN), Excluder (W.L. Gore and Associates, Inc., Flagstaff, AZ), Zenith (Cook, Inc., Bloomington, IN), and PowerLink (Endologix, Inc., Irvine, CA). The Ancure device is no longer FDA approved.

The present chapter serves as a brief introduction to the four clinically available devices and includes the anatomical algorithms we have used for device selection. Each device and its clinical results are discussed fully in subsequent chapters. The Ancure device has been withdrawn from clinical use for reasons related to the delivery system rather than to the endovascular graft itself. Therefore, although the Ancure device is no longer commercially available but was used widely before withdrawal, a knowledge of its construction and configuration may be useful when planning secondary interventions for implanted devices.

## Ancure device

There were three commercially available configurations of the Ancure device: tube, bifurcated, and aortoiliac. The bifurcated graft was used most frequently. All devices were unibody, unsupported woven polyester with proximal and distal attachment sites (Figure 8.1). The attachment sites were made of Elgiloy (Elgiloy Specialty Metals, Elgin, IL) and consisted of a Z frame with four V-shaped double hooks. The attachment system was hand sutured to the graft. The lateral edges of the graft had radiopaque markers to facilitate visualization during implantation and follow-up.

## Development

EndoVascular Technologies, acquired by Guidant Corporation in 1997, was founded in 1989 to develop an endovascular stent graft for repair of abdom-

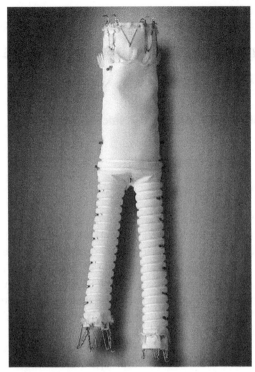

**Figure 8.1** The bifurcated Ancure stent graft (Guidant Corp.).

inal aortic aneurysms [2]. The initial device was a tube graft modeled after the work of Dr Harrison Lazarus, who in the 1980s placed polyester tube grafts into sheep. The company added bifurcated and aorto-uni-iliac devices in 1994 [2].

In 1993, Dr Wesley Moore was the first to use the device in clinical practice. This was the first commercially manufactured device to enter clinical trials in the United States. After modification of the deployment system, the device entered phase 3 clinical trials in 1998. Data from patients in phase 2 trials and from 89 patients in phase 3 trials were presented to the FDA in June 1999.

### Deployment

The Ancure device required surgical access to both femoral arteries. Snaring of the contralateral limb "pull wire" allowed the deployment of the unibody bifurcated device. The graft was delivered through a 25F introducer sheath and was unjacketed with both limbs above the aortic bifurcation. The graft was then pulled into position from both limbs. The proximal and distal hooks were secured by balloon dilatation.

## Clinical results

In the phase 1 clinical trial, most patients were treated with the tube graft and the first-generation attachment system. From 1993 to 1995, 102 patients received tubes and 12 received bifurcated grafts. Migration and endoleak occurred in several cases, requiring conversion to open repair [2]. In four cases the aneurysms had ruptured.

The phase 2 trial compared 111 open repairs with 153 tube, 268 bifurcated, and 121 aortoiliac grafts. Technical success was >90%. The aneurysm diameter had decreased at least 5 mm in 51.3% of the bifurcated grafts at 12 months and in 68.5% at 24 months. Of the bifurcated grafts, however, 2.1% had expanded >5 mm at 12 months and 1.1% had expanded >5 mm at 24 months. There have been no ruptures, and there were three late conversions to open repair.

The phase 3 trials began in 1998 and continued enrollment until FDA approval in September 1999. For the 290 bifurcated and 41 tube grafts placed, initial technical success was 94% [2]. The duration of hospital stay was decreased to 2 days, and both cardiac and pulmonary complications were fewer than in the phase 2 trials [2]. The endoleak rate, largely from type II endoleak, stayed relatively constant: 30% at 12 months and 23% at 24 months. There have been no ruptures since the attachment system was revised in 1995.

Because the Ancure device was an unsupported graft with only proximal and distal attachments, there were problems with limb obstruction. Iliac limb obstruction may be secondary to twisting or kinking of the limbs or to external compression, resulting in thrombosis.

With improved intraoperative detection using intravascular ultrasonography and intraoperative placement of a Wallstent venous endoprosthesis (Boston Scientific Corp., Natick, MA) in the iliac limbs, only 2 of the first 77 patients in the phase 3 trial required postoperative intervention [2]. The purported advantage of an unsupported graft was better accommodation of aortic remodeling after endograft placement. In the United States, more than 3000 Ancure devices were placed with favorable results overall.

## AneuRx device

The AneuRx device is a self-expanding, fully supported graft of woven polyester. The graft is attached by >2500 polyester sutures to a nickel-titanium (nitinol) exoskeleton (Figure 8.2). Currently, only a bifurcated configuration is available. The device is modular, with the longer limb measuring 16.5 cm and the shorter measuring 13.5 cm. Iliac extensions are available in diameters of 12, 13, 14, 15, and 16 mm in a standard length of 5.5 cm. Proximal extensions are available in diameters of 20, 22, 24, 26, and 28 mm in a standard length of 3.75 cm.

### Development

The AneuRx stent graft was designed by Dr Thomas J. Fogarty in 1993 [3]. AneuRx, Inc. (Sunnyvale, CA) was subsequently created, and the company

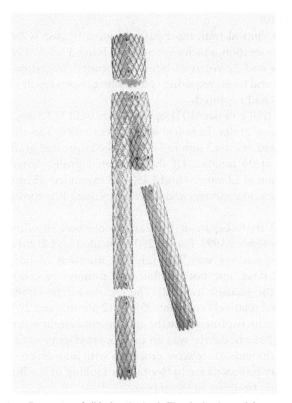

**Figure 8.2** The AneuRx stent graft (Medtronic, Inc.). The device is modular.

continued development of the graft. In 1995, animal studies were conducted at both Stanford University and Harbor-UCLA Medical Center. In 1996, Dr Rodney White was the first to use the device in clinical practice.

## Deployment

The AneuRx device main body and proximal extensions are preloaded in a 21F delivery sheath. The iliac limbs and extensions are preloaded in a 16F delivery sheath. Initially, these devices had blunt-tip sheaths; therefore, it had been our practice to first place a tapered sheath: a 22F Keller-Timmerman sheath for the main body (Cook, Inc.) and a 16F tapered sheath with radiopaque marker (Cook, Inc.) for contralateral limb deployment. This simplified navigation of the delivery sheaths. More recently, the delivery system was modified to include a long tapered-tip sheath, which obviates the need for an introducer sheath. A nose cone orientation marker and radiopaque markers on the stent graft allow axial and longitudinal orientation of the endograft under fluoroscopy. After the correct orientation is achieved, the base of the delivery sheath is marked and care is taken not to rotate the sheath during insertion, especially when small or tortuous iliac arteries are traversed. Placement occurs by self-expansion of the graft after removal of the covering sheath. It is our practice routinely to perform balloon angioplasty to profile with a 33-mm latex balloon (Boston Scientific Corp.) at the proximal, distal, and contralateral attachment sites and where the contralateral limb overlaps the main body of the device or the gate.

## Clinical results

Phase 1 trials began in June 1996 with 40 patients. Phase 2 trials enrolled 424 stent graft patients and 66 open surgical controls. Phase 3 trials enrolled 641 patients. In phase 2 and phase 3 trials, an additional 87 grafts were placed in high-risk patients, for a total of 1192 stent graft patients in all phases.

A 4-year clinical experience in the United States has been published [3]. Initial technical success was 98%, overall mortality was 10%, and 10 patients (0.8%) experienced aneurysmal rupture. Conversion to open repair occurred in 2.8% of the patients. Other secondary procedures were required in 8%.

As compared with open surgical controls, in the AneuRx group major morbidity was 50% less, operative blood loss was 60% less, and the duration of hospital stay was considerably shorter (3.4 vs 9.3 days).

At hospital dismissal, endoleaks, largely type II, were reported in 38–50% of the patients who received an AneuRx device. At 1 month, this number decreased to 13%. Investigators have found that the presence of an endoleak at 1 month increased the likelihood of aneurysmal expansion but did not affect patient survival, rupture rate, conversion to open repair, occurrence of a new endoleak, or stent graft migration. Worldwide, more than 10 000 AneuRx devices have been placed with overall favorable results.

In December 2003, the FDA Center for Devices and Radiological Health [4] published an update on mortality associated with the AneuRx device. The findings were from a cohort of 942 patients who initially received the device during premarket study. Analyses of the Excluder and Zenith devices were not included because long-term data for them were not available. The perioperative mortality for the AneuRx device was 1.5% (14 of 942 patients). There were 8 aneurysm-related deaths during the 3-year follow-up period, which covered 2080 patient-years. The annualized mortality rate was 0.40%. At 3 years after implantation, the estimated aneurysm-related death rate was 2.7%. This underscores the importance of patient selection, including surgical risk and life expectancy, for EVAR, regardless of the device. We have had excellent results with over 100 AneuRx devices.

## Excluder device

In November 2002, the Excluder bifurcated endoprosthesis was approved for clinical use by the FDA. It is the only endovascular device consisting of expanded polytetrafluoroethylene (ePTFE) and a fully supported nitinol exoskeleton (Figure 8.3). The ePTFE is bonded to the nitinol without sutures.

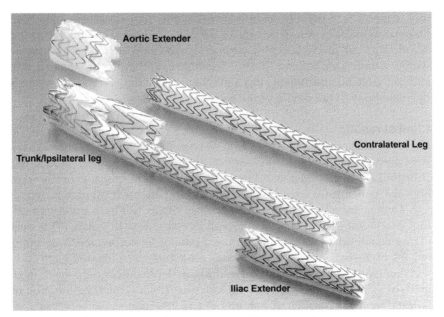

**Figure 8.3** The Excluder bifurcated endoprosthesis (W.L. Gore and Associates, Inc.).

This modular device has a minimum of two components, with iliac and aortic extensions.

### Development
In 1995, W.L. Gore and Associates, Inc., began development of the Excluder device. It became commercially available outside the United States in 1997. Between the fall of 1997 and the summer of 2003, >8500 patients worldwide were treated with this device. Initial results were first reported by Semba *et al.* [5].

### Deployment
The proximal graft diameter ranges from 23 to 28.5 mm. The distal diameter ranges from 12 to 14.5 mm for the ipsilateral iliac limb and up to 20 mm for the contralateral limb. The main body is introduced with an 18F sheath, and the iliac components are preloaded in a 12F sheath. The deployment system consists of the device mounted on an ePTFE sleeve. The device is released using the SIM-PULL deployment system (W.L. Gore and Associates, Inc.).

### Clinical results
The final clinical trial data for the Excluder bifurcated device were presented to the FDA on September 9, 2002. On the basis of those data, the device received conditional approval. Since then, the device has been implanted in 12 000 patients worldwide with limited follow-up.

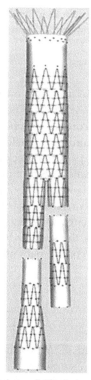

**Figure 8.4** The Zenith AAA endovascular graft (Cook, Inc.).

## Zenith device

The Zenith AAA endovascular graft consists of a woven polyester graft supported with stainless steel Z stents. The device is currently available in a bifurcated configuration (Figure 8.4).

### Development

The current Zenith device is the end result of several Dacron (DuPont, Wilmington, DE) graft and stainless steel prototypes. These include the Ivancev-Malmö (Cook, Inc.) and Chuter (Cook, Inc.) devices. Modifications include proximal barbs and hooks and both proximal and distal trigger wires, which allow for extremely accurate deployment. The current device is constructed of full-thickness woven polyester fabric sewn to self-expanding stainless steel Z stents with braided polyester and polypropylene monofilament sutures. The bare suprarenal stent contains barbs at 3-mm increments. Gold markers facilitate orientation of the device.

### Deployment

The main body delivery system is either 18F or 20F, depending on the device diameter. As mentioned previously, proximal and distal trigger wires affix the device to the delivery system. The iliac graft components are preloaded in either a 14F or 16F delivery system. All components are compatible with a 0.035-inch wire guide.

## Clinical results

The Zenith device received FDA approval on June 12, 2002, which followed widespread use in Europe and Australia. The US clinical study was a multicenter, nonrandomized study comparing open aneurysm repair with high- and standard-risk EVAR. Anatomical exclusions from EVAR were circumferential proximal neck thrombus, proximal neck length <15 mm, proximal neck diameter (outer wall to outer wall) <18 mm or >28 mm, severe neck angulation (>60°), and iliac artery diameter <7.5 mm. At 1-year follow-up after EVAR, aneurysmal rupture occurred in 1% of the high-risk patients and in none of the standard-risk patients. One-year mortality was 9% among the high-risk patients, 3.5% among the standard-risk patients, and 3.8% among the standard-risk open surgical control patients. We have had excellent results with 51 Zenith devices.

## PowerLink device

### Development

The PowerLink device received FDA postmarket approval on October 29, 2004. The device has a unique "single-wire" design and a cobalt-chromium alloy "cage" that is covered with polytetrafluoroethylene. It is available in a bifurcated design (Figure 8.5).

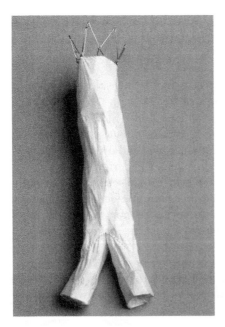

**Figure 8.5** The PowerLink stent graft (Endologix, Inc.).

## Deployment

The device requires a proximal aortic neck length of at least 15 mm and a diameter between 18 and 26 mm. Iliac fixation requires a length of at least 15 mm and a diameter between 10 and 14 mm. The main body of the device is deployed with a 21F delivery system. The device is currently available in a length of 80 or 100 mm and a proximal graft diameter of 25 or 28 mm.

## Clinical results

A prospective controlled multicenter trial from 15 sites included 192 experimental and 66 control patients. Technical success was achieved in 97.9%. There was a single procedure-related death. Secondary procedures were required in 10% of the patients, for either endoleak or limb obstruction [6]. A decrease in sac diameter and proximal neck angulation has also been reported in a retrospective review [7].

## Device selection

Preoperative imaging is the cornerstone of patient and device selection. This is discussed in detail elsewhere in this book (see Chapter 3).

As experience is gained with EVAR, many of the circumstances initially thought to be absolute anatomical exclusion criteria for endograft placement have become relative. For instance, iliofemoral access is optimal if the vessels have minimal tortuosity and calcification, with a minimal diameter of 7.5 mm. In our experience, however, with the availability of hydrophilic tapered dilators and the Lunderquist guidewire (Cook, Inc.), the majority of suboptimal iliac arteries have been traversed with the chosen device. In our practice, though, circumferential calcification of a small vessel continues to be a contraindication to endovascular repair. When hydrophilic dilators fail to provide an optimal result, the alternatives are (1) placement of a prosthetic conduit from the common iliac artery proximally and tunneled to the groin, (2) placement of an aorto-uni-iliac device (assuming one iliofemoral system can be traversed), and (3) placement of a femorofemoral bypass graft after occlusion of the contralateral common iliac artery.

When the caliber and extent of calcification are equal in both iliofemoral segments, we prefer to place the component requiring the larger introducer sheath through the femoral artery ipsilateral to the major aneurysmal thrombus burden. This may prevent "snowplowing" of thrombi into the visceral aorta as the tip of the sheath is advanced proximally.

Common iliac artery diameters larger than 13.4 mm for the Ancure device and 16 mm for the AneuRx device do not allow for a distal seal. The additional maneuvers required may include relocation of the iliac bifurcation to allow for a suitable distal landing zone [8]; unilateral or bilateral hypogastric artery embolization and extension of the stent graft to the external iliac artery; or construction of a "distal flare" of the limb. Each alternative is discussed elsewhere in this book (see Chapter 21).

**Table 8.1** Characteristics of commercially available bifurcated devices.

| Characteristic | AneuRx* | Excluder[†] | Zenith[‡] | PowerLink[§] |
|---|---|---|---|---|
| Maximal device diameter, mm | | | | |
|     Proximal | 28 | 28.5 | 32 | 28 |
|     Distal | 16 | 14.5–20 | 22 | 20[ǁ] |
| Introducer sheath diameter, French | | | | |
|     Main body | 21 | 18 | 18–20 | 21 |
|     Contralateral | 16 | 12 | 14–16 | 12 |
| Minimal proximal neck length, mm | 15 | 15 | 15 | 15 |
| Minimal iliac attachment site length, mm | 10 | 10 | 14 | 15 |

*Medtronic, Inc.
[†]W.L. Gore and Associates, Inc.
[‡]Cook, Inc.
[§]Endologix, Inc.
[ǁ]Requires distal limb extension.

**Table 8.2** Algorithm for selection of endovascular devices according to the diameter of the proximal neck of the aorta.*

| | Proximal neck diameter, mm | | |
|---|---|---|---|
| Device | ≤25 | >25–28 | >28–32 |
| AneuRx[†] | Yes | – | – |
| Excluder[‡] | Yes | – | – |
| Talent[†] | Yes | Yes | Yes |
| Zenith[§] | Yes | Yes | – |
| PowerLink[ǁ] | Yes | – | – |

*Devices require a proximal aortic neck length of at least 15 mm, except the Talent device, which requires at least 10 mm.
[†]Medtronic, Inc.
[‡]W.L. Gore and Associates, Inc.
[§]Cook, Inc.
[ǁ]Endologix, Inc.

Proximal neck angulation (that is, the angle of the proximal neck relative to the long axis of the aneurysm) of >60° has led to a decrease in the durability of the AneuRx device [9]. Severe angulation with a proximal type I endoleak or with continued aneurysmal growth requires conversion to an open procedure.

Table 8.1 summarizes the characteristics of the currently available FDA-approved bifurcated devices. Tables 8.2 and 8.3 show our algorithms for the selection of endovascular devices according to aortic and iliac diameters. The Talent aortic endograft (Medtronic, Inc.) is included because, although not FDA approved, this device offers considerable flexibility in endograft placement. Our experience with 22 devices has been rewarding.

**Table 8.3** Algorithm for selection of endovascular devices according to the diameter of the common iliac artery.

| Device | Common iliac diameter, mm | |
|---|---|---|
| | ≤14 | >14–20 |
| AneuRx* | Yes | – |
| Excluder† | Yes | – |
| Talent* | Yes | Yes |
| Zenith‡ | Yes | Yes |
| PowerLink§ | Yes | Yes‖ |

*Medtronic, Inc.
†W.L. Gore and Associates, Inc.
‡Cook, Inc.
§Endologix, Inc.
‖Distal graft diameter can be increased with a 20 × 55-mm limb extension.

## Conclusion

When EVAR is planned, consideration of the optimal device is based on aortic and iliac anatomical features. At present, no device uniformly offers an acceptable proximal seal when the proximal neck angulation is >60° or the neck is conical (10% increase in neck diameter from the infrarenal aorta to the distal neck).

The four currently available devices differ in fabric and construction. In addition, delivery system diameter and maximal graft diameter are considerations for device selection. Because long-term data are available only for the AneuRx device, further clinical surveillance may elucidate the value or weaknesses of the other devices.

## References

1 Parodi JC, Palmaz JC, Barone HD. Transfemoral intraluminal graft implantation for abdominal aortic aneurysms. *Ann Vasc Surg* 1991; **5**: 491–9.

2 Makaroun MS. The Ancure endografting system: an update. *J Vasc Surg* 2001; **33**(Suppl): S129–34.

3 Zarins CK, White RA, Moll FL *et al.* The AneuRx stent graft: four-year results and worldwide experience 2000. *J Vasc Surg* 2001; **33**(Suppl): S136–45; published erratum in *J Vasc Surg* 2001; **33**: 1318.

4 US Food and Drug Administration. FDA public health notification: updated data on mortality associated with Medtronic AVE AneuRx stent graft system. December 17, 2003. Available at: http://www.fda.gov/cdrh/safety/aneurx.html. Accessed July 12, 2004.

5 Semba CP, Dake MD, Razavi MK *et al.* Abdominal aortic aneurysm repair with the W. L. Gore Excluder endovascular stent-graft: technique and potential pitfalls. *Tech Vasc Intervent Radiol* 1999; **2**: 127–32.

6 Carpenter JP, the Endologix Investigators. Midterm results of the multicenter trial of the PowerLink bifurcated system for endovascular aortic aneurysm repair. *J Vasc Surg* 2004; **40**: 849–59.

7 White R. Sac remodeling with the PowerLink stent graft for AAA. Presented at the International Society for Endovascular Therapy, January 25–29, 2005, Miami, FL.

8 Parodi JC, Ferreira M. Relocation of the iliac artery bifurcation to facilitate endoluminal treatment of abdominal aortic aneurysms. *J Endovasc Surg* 1999; **6**: 342–7.

9 Sternbergh WC III, Carter G, York JW, Yoselevitz M, Money SR. Aortic neck angulation predicts adverse outcome with endovascular abdominal aortic aneurysm repair. *J Vasc Surg* 2002; **35**: 482–6.

# CHAPTER 9

# Ancure endograft

## Thomas C. Naslund, MD

### Introduction

The Ancure endograft (Guidant Corp., Menlo Park, CA) had its genesis from a patent filed by Harrison Lazarus in 1988 [1]. The idea was to design a synthetic surgical graft with Z stent, self-expanding attachment systems sutured to either end of the prosthesis. These attachment systems had hooks to allow fixation of the prosthesis to the arterial wall (Figure 9.1). This constituted the patent that was approved and later acquired by a venture capital company, EndoVascular Technologies, Inc. (EVT).

EVT refined the tube endovascular graft as well as multiple deployment systems to place the prosthesis within the human aorta. The first clinical implant of the EVT graft was performed by Wesley Moore at the University of California, Los Angeles, in February 1993 [2]. Subsequent development of a bifurcated prosthesis was undertaken, again with multiple deployment systems. In 1997, during phase 3 clinical trials, the Guidant Corporation acquired EVT. In the fall of 1999, Guidant completed the clinical study and obtained US Food and Drug Administration (FDA) approval of the Ancure tube and bifurcated endografts.

### Design

The uniqueness of the Ancure endograft, compared with other endovascular grafts, is obvious at first inspection. It is a woven Dacron graft (DuPont, Wilmington, DE), similar to surgical grafts, that is sutured to attachment systems with a Z stent design. Hooks on the stent struts provide fixation to the native arterial wall. In addition, two rows of radiopaque metallic reference marks are positioned 180° from each other for radiographic assessment of orientation during deployment and late follow-up.

The Ancure endograft has a unibody design; there are no modular connections. In this respect, it most closely resembles a surgical graft after implantation. It is flexible like a surgical graft and it accommodates positional changes owing to arterial remodeling as the size of the aneurysm changes. Because it has a unibody design, there are no components to separate or permit leakage of blood from the prosthesis. Attachment systems and hooks that penetrate the arterial wall hold the prosthesis in position. There is no sup-

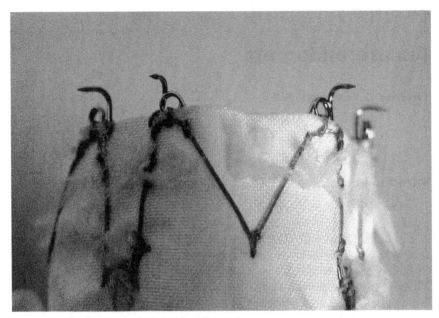

**Figure 9.1** Attachment system with hooks as depicted in the patent filed by Lazarus (1).

porting exoskeleton or columnar strength in the body of the prosthesis to provide either a friction seal of the prosthesis against the native arterial wall or resistance to shortening.

Three types of Ancure endografts are available. The tube, bifurcated, and aorto-uni-iliac endografts are designed for the various anatomical configurations of aneurysms and their associated iliac artery anatomical features and diseases (Figure 9.2).

The bifurcated endograft provides the most versatility. It can be used with or without a distal aortic neck, it allows deployment distal to iliac aneurysms in some patients, and it is remarkably durable. After the implantation procedure for the bifurcated endograft is mastered, deployment of the tube endograft or the aorto-uni-iliac endograft is exceedingly easy.

The tube endograft can be used when a good distal neck and ectatic iliac arteries make a bifurcated endograft less desirable. It can also be used if the surgeon wants to treat patients who have normal iliac arteries and a distal neck. I prefer to limit the use of the tube endograft in favor of the bifurcated endograft wherever possible. This bias results from concern about deterioration of the distal neck or the possibility of a distal leak, which could be eliminated with use of the bifurcated endograft. I have a single case experience of using this endograft in a thoracic aneurysm with good outcome. It is rare, however, that a patient with a thoracic aortic aneurysm has an aortic diame-

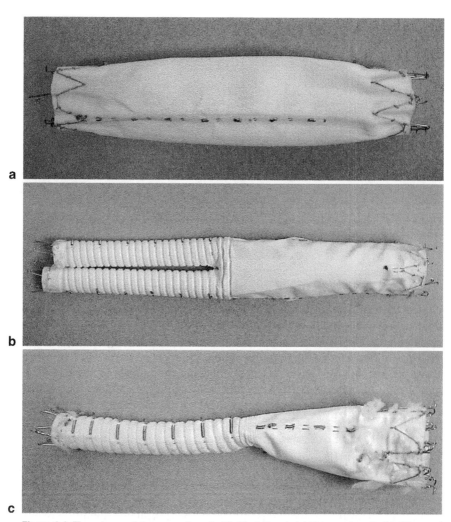

**Figure 9.2** Three types of Ancure endografts (Guidant Corp.). (a) Tube endograft. (b) Bifurcated endograft. (c) Aorto-uni-iliac endograft.

ter sufficiently small or a duration of disease sufficiently short for this device to be considered.

The aorto-uni-iliac endograft allows easy treatment of patients who have one iliac artery that is either occluded, severely tortuous, or stenotic. Additionally, it is useful for a small-diameter distal neck that is unsuitable for attachment of a tube endograft and too narrow for a bifurcated endograft. Use of the aorto-uni-iliac endograft is coupled with intentional contralateral iliac occlusion with an endovascular occlusion device or surgical ligation. A femorofemoral bypass completes the procedure.

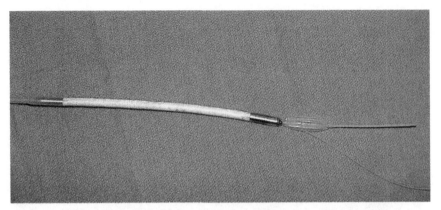

**Figure 9.3** A delivery catheter includes a compressed endovascular graft housed within the jacket, a contralateral pull wire, and a balloon.

The delivery system for the Ancure endograft has been simplified through clinical trials and again at market release. The compressed endograft is delivered within a single 23F delivery catheter, which is an over-the-wire endoluminal device. The balloon used for full expansion and seating of the proximal attachment hooks is on the tip of the delivery catheter (Figure 9.3). The bifurcated prosthesis has a wire affixed to a locking mechanism in the contralateral limb. The wire exits from the tip of the delivery catheter and allows for control of the position and deployment of the contralateral limb of the endograft.

## Implantation

Deployment of the bifurcated endovascular prosthesis occurs in a stepwise fashion. Arteriography with a reference-marked catheter is useful either preoperatively or at the time of graft implantation. This allows definition of any important arterial occlusive lesions in the iliac or renal arteries as well as measurement of the length of the prosthesis needed.

**1** A 27F sheath is first introduced into the ipsilateral iliac artery. The 27F Guidant sheath has a double hemostatic valve with space to allow the introduction of variously sized devices while maintaining hemostasis (Figure 9.4).

**2** The pull wire attached to the contralateral limb of the bifurcated endograft is introduced through the sheath and captured with a snare in the abdominal aorta which was introduced through the contralateral femoral access.

**3** The pull wire is withdrawn through the contralateral common femoral access and is used to control the contralateral limb.

**4** The delivery catheter is then advanced into the aorta, a plastic jacket that covers the prosthesis is withdrawn, and the proximal attachment system is appropriately positioned with radiographic guidance.

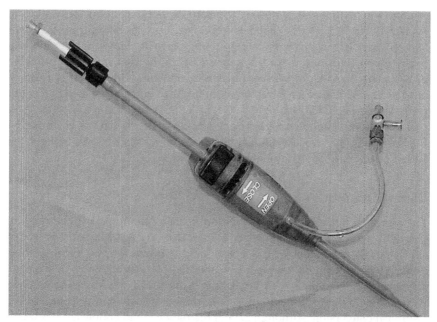

**Figure 9.4** A 27F sheath with a double hemostatic valve that maintains hemostasis during the introduction of devices of various sizes.

**5** The proximal attachment system is deployed by a simple pull wire with nearly pinpoint accuracy.
**6** The balloon for expansion of the proximal attachment is positioned across the proximal attachment and inflated.
**7** The pull wire attached to the contralateral limb is used as access to place a torque catheter that engages the contralateral limb and allows manipulation of the limb, either proximally or distally, as well as torque of the limb, if needed, for appropriate orientation.
**8** After it is positioned radiographically, the contralateral limb is deployed and the hooks from the attachment system are embedded in the arterial wall by using balloon inflations.
**9** The ipsilateral limb is positioned and deployed by using a pull wire, after which the delivery catheter is removed.
**10** Balloon inflations within the ipsilateral limb allow seating of the attachment system into the native arterial wall.
**11** Arteriography completes the procedure.

The kissing-balloon technique is used with high-pressure (8 atm, 808 kPa) inflations in the iliac endograft limbs to weaken the native arterial wall, permitting maximal limb expansion and limiting extrinsic limb compression. With this technique, minor defects in endograft limbs on completion angiography are not pursued with stents, whereas kinks or compression at iliac origins or in tortuous segments are treated with self-expanding stents that are oversized in relation to the limb being stented. Intravascular ultrasonography is used sparingly in favor of stenting if angiography demonstrates any limb compression that may place the patency of the limb at risk. It is probably important to avoid high-pressure inflation of balloons within the distal attachment systems because such treatment invites iliac injury in an area that is not protected by an endograft.

Deployment of tube endografts or aorto-uni-iliac endografts is simple by comparison: only proximal and distal deployments are needed, without the added complexity of a contralateral limb.

## Clinical results

The phase 2 clinical results from the bifurcated Ancure endograft compare favorably with outcomes for other devices. Among the 242 patients in this clinical trial, one patient experienced device migration; no ruptures had occurred at a mean follow-up of 36 months [3]. Additionally, at 3 years, aneurysm size had decreased by at least 5 mm in 74% of the patients. Two patients had a fractured hook in the attachment system, and 2% underwent a surgical conversion. Although 27% of the patients had endoleaks at 3 years, aneurysm size decreased in 35% of the patients with leaks. Type I endoleaks existed in nearly 4% of the patients at 1 year but had been eliminated by 3 years, leaving only type II and indeterminate type leaks. Endograft limb interventions occurred in 50 of the 242 patients; 34 of these were performed in the first 12 months. About half of the limb interventions were for endoleak and half for decreased limb blood flow.

In a personal experience with 130 Ancure endografts with follow-up of 1 or more years, similar results were seen with no migration or rupture. Aneurysm sac diameter decreased in 56% of the patients at 1 year, 71% at 3 years, and 100% at 4 or more years of follow-up. Endoleaks were identified in 25% of the patients. Curiously, only three patients had postoperative intervention for decreased endograft limb blood flow. The most likely cause was aggressive angioplasty of endograft limbs rather than intralimb stent placement, which was done in only 14% of the patients. Two patients had an intraoperative surgical conversion and one had a late surgical conversion (for infection).

The remarkably low risk of migration and the freedom from rupture with the Ancure endograft make the long-term results enviable by any standard. Nonetheless, durability—specifically, endovascular leak and decreased endograft limb blood flow—is a weakness of this and other endovascular prostheses when compared with conventional open surgery.

## Troubleshooting

Some endovascular surgeons, usually those with limited Ancure endograft experience, find Ancure endografts more difficult to implant than other devices. Although the Ancure endograft may seem more difficult to use until the implantation procedure is completely mastered, the freedom from migration and rupture afforded by this endograft continues to make it an attractive choice for endovascular aneurysm repair.

Several predictable points of difficulty during deployment can be negotiated successfully with appropriate planning and a full knowledge of bailout techniques. The most likely causes of difficulty in placing the Ancure endograft are sheath placement, wire wraps, resistance to jacket movement, wire trapped on hooks, contralateral wire advancement, negotiating tortuous iliac vessels, and failure to remove the delivery catheter. By prospectively recognizing these potential problems and making deployment adjustments, a difficult and time-consuming deployment or even a conversion may be avoided.

The 27F sheath is ideally placed in the common iliac artery. When the sheath does not advance to the common iliac artery, however, a successful operation can still be accomplished by leaving the sheath (preferably one 15 cm long) in the external iliac artery. Alternatively, the graft can be placed without a sheath, commonly termed "bareback." Furthermore, if the sheath or device cannot pass the external iliac artery, an extraperitoneal approach permits suturing of a synthetic graft to the common iliac artery and creating a conduit through which a sheath can be inserted and the graft implanted. The added support from extra-stiff guidewires helps in gaining sheath access by helping to straighten the course traversed by the sheath. Sequential dilations of the iliac artery can be accomplished with success, but the risk of arterial injury must be appreciated.

The contralateral wire wraps around the ipsilateral wire during about 50% of the procedures involving the bifurcated Ancure endograft. This is easily recognized when the delivery catheter reaches the aortic bifurcation and is remedied either by removing the delivery catheter and rotating it 360° or by inserting the delivery catheter as far as possible and providing 360° rotation while moving the catheter up and down within the aorta. This motion allows the rotation to be translated throughout the length of the delivery catheter. After the surgeon is certain that the wire wrap has been eliminated (Figure 9.5), the device can be positioned and deployed without concern of a twist in the trunk of the prosthesis.

When the jacket is withdrawn, resistance ("jacket lock") can be encountered if the device is in a curved or bent configuration near the distal end of the endograft limbs. Resistance to jacket movement can be minimized by advancing the device in an effort to eliminate or minimize any bend at this point along with injection of heparinized saline through the flush port at the time of withdrawing the jacket.

If gentle tension on the contralateral pull wire is not maintained while the jacket is withdrawn, this wire can loop over the exposed hooks of the proximal attachment and become trapped. Advancing the wire and creating a large loop frequently allows the wire to slide off the hooks. If this simple maneuver fails, placement of a guide catheter, 8F or larger, over the pull wire can assist in manipulating the wire off the hooks. Additionally, inflation of the

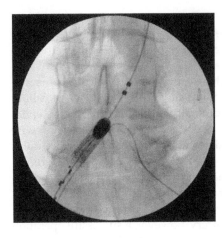

**Figure 9.5** Appropriate insertion without the contralateral wire wrapping around the ipsilateral wire at the level of the aortic bifurcation.

aortic balloon helps move the proximal portion of the device, creating additional space to permit the wire to pass by the exposed hooks. Similarly, withdrawing the stiff wire from the proximal portion of the device induces movement at the tip.

Contralateral limb deployment may be associated with resistance to advancing the contralateral wire into the body of the endograft. A lock ball on the wire serves as an impediment to wire advancement. This wire advancement is needed to introduce a balloon catheter to seat the contralateral limb and its attachment system. Deflation of the aortic balloon, allowing the endograft limb to fill with pulsatile flow, helps open the endograft and allow wire advancement. When the wire will not advance, however, an 8F guide catheter placed over the wire and inserted to the end of the contralateral limb permits a second access with a hydrophilic wire introduced through the endograft limb, thereby permitting balloon dilatation.

Perhaps most importantly, difficulties must be expected in the presence of iliac occlusive lesions or tortuosity. In such cases a combination of predeployment iliac angioplasty and the use of a stiff wire in the contralateral iliac artery during endograft limb deployment helps minimize the risk that intrinsic arterial disease will prevent endograft expansion.

The presence of tortuous iliac arteries does not prevent the use of an Ancure endograft but can require the use of an extra-stiff wire adjacent to the contralateral limb, so that the native vessel remains as straight as possible during deployment and contralateral wire advancement. If needed, particularly with occlusive disease, angioplasty performed outside the endolimb over this stiff wire can assist in allowing endograft expansion and advancement of the contralateral wire.

Another predictable procedural problem is the inability to remove the delivery catheter after completing endograft deployment. This can be expected if the ipsilateral iliac artery has notable atherosclerosis and has not been dilated or if there is tortuosity or subtotal expansion of the ipsilateral attachment. Usually the ipsilateral limb can be expanded sufficiently to withdraw the delivery catheter if the following steps are taken: applying moderate force, rotating the aortic balloon handle, and inflating and deflating the contralateral iliac limb balloon opposite the area where the proximal capsule is engaging the ipsilateral limb. In the rare circumstances when these maneuvers are not successful, the access wire is removed, the delivery catheter is transected with a wire or pin cutter, and all the components of the delivery catheter are withdrawn except the balloon shaft, which is joined to the 23F proximal capsule. A wire can be replaced and the balloon shaft can be pulled and manipulated more easily to allow removal. If this also fails, a 10F or larger sheath is placed over the balloon shaft and advanced as far as possible, allowing secondary access with a hydrophilic wire placed into the ipsilateral endograft limb. The limb is expanded with balloon inflations, allowing removal of the remainder of the delivery catheter.

## Attachment fixation

Most other prostheses that have been in clinical studies and clinical use are modular devices without a firm mechanical fixation to the arterial wall. Instead, a friction seal from the radial strength of the prosthesis provides attachment to the arterial wall. Reports have suggested that migration of such devices occurs in various percentages of patients treated [4–6]. More recently, devices in feasibility trials have a degree of mechanical fixation, clearly an attempt to avoid migration risks. The Ancure endograft, although the first of its kind, was developed with a key component that prevents migration, at least in the intermediate-term follow-up available thus far. It remains to be seen whether long-term results of at least a decade will show that migration risks are greater than currently defined. Although decreased limb blood flow and thrombosis risks have been reported to be of concern with the Ancure endograft, my experience is that these detrimental outcomes are unusual. Others may disagree, but I feel that these complications are technique dependent, at least to some degree.

## Limitations

The design of the Ancure endograft does not easily lend itself to the management of concomitant iliac artery aneurysms. Nonetheless, one limb can be deployed in an external iliac artery distal to the internal iliac artery. Endografts are available with various combinations of limb lengths, and the hope is that even more combinations will be manufactured in the future.

Use of the Ancure bifurcated endograft in the iliac arteries is limited in part because the limb diameters are half the diameter of the aortic trunk. This configuration does not always result in an ideal match in size between the iliac arteries and the aortic neck. In some patients, the aortic trunk is intentionally oversized to allow an adequate diameter of the iliac limbs. In other patients, particularly those in which the external iliac artery is planned as a landing site, the diameter of the iliac limb in the external iliac artery is larger than desired. A broader selection of products in the future may solve some of these technical shortcomings.

Another notable shortcoming is access size. The 23F delivery system is difficult to place in the aorta in some patients, including small women and men, particularly those with substantial iliac artery atherosclerosis. Nonetheless, it is uncommon for me to identify patients who are not candidates for the Ancure endograft because of the diameter of the external iliac artery. Either the use of a technique involving dilatation of the external iliac artery (when atherosclerosis is not prominent) or the use of an arterial conduit directly to the common iliac artery allows the prosthesis to be used in virtually all patients suitable for endovascular repair, thereby providing the low risk of migration and rupture that would be expected from the use of the Ancure endograft.

The complexity of deployment of the Ancure endograft has frequently been discussed. It is true that placement of this prosthesis, rather than a modular prosthesis, requires a higher level of endovascular skill, but after the skill is acquired, the prosthesis is not difficult to place. The benefits from the prosthesis tend to outweigh the issue of having to acquire additional endovascular skills. Furthermore, the development of advanced skills strengthens the endovascular surgeon's technique for other endovascular procedures.

## The recall

In spring 2001, the Guidant Corporation voluntarily recalled its Ancure tube and bifurcated endografts. The rationale behind this recall was largely regulatory. Concern was raised that the risk of deployment complications may not be the same as in clinical trials. Also, advanced techniques used in training courses as well as techniques advocated by corporate support teams were not listed in the instructions for use provided in the device label.

Discussions between Guidant and the FDA resulted in the design of a trial in which intraoperative deployment complications and their remedies were monitored. The intent was to demonstrate that alterations in deployment techniques that evolved since marketing began, as well as the complications during deployment, mirror those of the clinical trials before FDA approval.

In August 2001, the FDA granted Guidant full market release of the Ancure endograft, and use resumed before the new trial was completed. The results of this trial demonstrated success rates similar to those of the premarket clinical trials [7].

By June 2003, the Guidant Ancure endograft had further problems: the US Department of Justice filed criminal charges against Guidant for failing to report a substantial number of postmarket operative complications that required federal reporting. Guidant settled with the Department of Justice, paid a large fine, and withdrew the Ancure endograft from the US market on October 1, 2003.

## Summary

For the repair of abdominal aortic aneurysms, the Guidant Ancure endograft provides a gratifyingly low risk of device migration, rupture, or late complication involving decreased limb blood flow. The technique of deployment may help decrease iliac limb difficulties in late follow-up and decrease the incidence of intraoperative deployment problems. Although other prostheses will undoubtedly enter the marketplace, only long-term results for patient outcome and freedom from rupture will determine whether such prostheses are superior to the Guidant Ancure endograft.

## References

1 Lazarus HM. Intraluminal graft device, system and method (1988 United States US Patent Number 4,787,899). Retrieved December 4, 2003, from the World Wide Web:http://patft.uspto.gov/netacgi/nph-Parser?Sect1=PTO2&Sect2=HITOFF&p=1&u=/netahtml/search-bool.html&r=1&f=G&1=50&col=AND&d=ptxt&s1=4787899.WKU.&OS=PN/4787899&RS=PN/4787899.

2 Moore WS, Vescera CL. Repair of abdominal aortic aneurysm by transfemoral endovascular graft placement. *Ann Surg* 1994; **220**: 331–9.

3 Makaroun M, Chaikof E, Naslund T, Matsumura J. Efficacy of the bifurcated Ancure endograft versus open repair of abdominal aortic aneurysms: a reappraisal. *J Vasc Surg* 2002; **35**: 203–10.

4 Zarins CK, White RA, Schwarten D *et al*. AneuRx stent graft versus open surgical repair of abdominal aortic aneurysms: multicenter prospective clinical trial. *J Vasc Surg* 1999; **29**: 292–305.

5 Zarins CK, White RA, Fogarty TJ. Aneurysm rupture after endovascular repair using the AneuRx stent graft. *J Vasc Surg* 2000; **31**: 960–70.

6 Cao P, Verzini F, Zannetti S *et al*. Device migration after endoluminal abdominal aortic aneurysm repair: analysis of 113 cases with a minimum follow-up period of 2 years. *J Vasc Surg* 2002; **35**: 229–35.

7 Naslund TC, Becker SY. Technical success from endovascular aneurysm repair in the post-marketing era: a multicenter prospective trial. *Ann Vasc Surg* 2003; **17**: 35–42. Epub Jan 15, 2003.

# CHAPTER 10

# AneuRx stent graft system

**John W. York, MD, Samuel R. Money, MD, FACS, MBA**

## Introduction

The open surgical treatment of abdominal aortic aneurysms (AAAs) has been performed successfully for more than 40 years with the goal of preventing aneurysmal rupture and death. Since the late 1980s, the shift toward less invasive surgical options for standard surgical disease has led to the development of alternative vascular surgical techniques for accomplishing this goal. The introduction of the endoluminal system for the repair of infrainguinal AAAs in 1991 was a milestone in vascular surgery. The development of this technique, although industry driven, progressed at an unprecedented pace from the initial reports to the approval by the US Food and Drug Administration (FDA) in 6 years. Although some have ardently embraced endovascular AAA repair, others view it without enthusiasm. This is primarily because of the limited long-term experience with the new technology as well as the associated complications that may be of great clinical significance. Although still relatively new, endovascular AAA repair has been shown to have results comparable to those of open AAA repair in terms of morbidity and mortality [1,2].

The AneuRx endovascular AAA repair system (Medtronic Inc., Minneapolis, MN) was granted FDA approval for commercial distribution in September 1999 and was the lone endovascular AAA device commercially available in the United States for a while. The current model is a modular bifurcated system constructed of woven polyester with a nitinol exoskeleton. This system, commercially available in the United States since only 1999, has been used in other countries since 1997. This chapter reviews the development of the AneuRx system and the current experience with the device.

## Historical perspective

The technique of surgical repair of large or symptomatic AAAs using transabdominal aortic exposure and transmural fixation of a prosthetic graft was first reported by Dubost et al. [3] in 1952 and has remained the standard of care for this form of aortic disease since then. None of the modifications to the technique, including retroperitoneal exposure and laparoscopic AAA repair, have been embraced as commonly used alternatives to transabdominal repair. The first report of an endoluminal AAA repair, however, in 1991 by Parodi *et al.* [4] ignited an explosion of focused investigation toward the development of a less invasive option for the surgical repair of AAAs.

The initial experiments with endoluminal exclusion of AAAs in animals began in 1976. The experimental endoluminal devices were handmade, constructed of a Dacron graft (DuPont, Wilmington, DE) sewn onto a Palmaz balloon-expandable stent (Cordis Corp., Miami, FL) at the proximal end. Artificial AAA models were constructed in experimental animals with a fusiform Dacron graft that was surgically interposed in the infrarenal aorta. These studies successfully demonstrated that the device could be delivered transfemorally with relatively low-profile sheaths. AAA exclusion was achieved as the Palmaz stent replaced transmural suture in fixing the proximal end of the graft to the aorta by frictional forces. Later experiments used an additional Palmaz stent at the distal end of the graft to achieve total exclusion of the AAA.

On the basis of these animal studies, the first-generation devices deployed in human subjects were tube endografts introduced under anesthesia into the aorta by retrograde cannulation of the common femoral artery with a 22F sheath. The report included the experience with five patients who were felt to be at high risk for open aortic surgery. Each device was custom-made, using standard stents and Dacron prosthetic grafts, to correspond anatomically to each patient (Figure 10.1). The device was successfully deployed in all patients

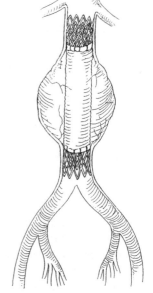

**Figure 10.1** The tube endograft first deployed in humans for the exclusion of abdominal aortic aneurysms by Parodi *et al.* [4] in 1991. (Reprinted from Parodi JC, Palmaz JC, Barone HD, Transfemoral intraluminal graft implantation for abdominal aortic aneurysms, *Ann Vasc Surg* 1991; **5**: 491–9, Copyright 1991, with permission of the International Society of Endovascular Specialists.)

and satisfactory exclusion of each AAA was documented at 3, 8, 9, and 12 months [4].

The tube endograft then evolved into the aorto-uni-iliac system: a lengthened tube endograft was extended into the common iliac artery, the contralateral iliac artery was occluded, and a femorofemoral bypass was used to reestablish contralateral lower extremity perfusion. This system alleviated problems associated with distal device attachment in the aorta and allowed for endoluminal repair for patients with AAAs that extended into the iliac artery.

Subsequently, this first-generation device was modified into a bifurcated system (EndoVascular Technologies, Inc., Menlo Park, CA) that used proximal and distal stent fixation. This system further widened the scope of patients who were candidates for endovascular repair by including those with bilateral iliac aneurysmal disease. This system also eliminated the requirement of iatrogenic occlusion of the contralateral iliac artery.

After 6 years of clinical trials and design improvements, two endovascular devices were approved for commercial use by the FDA in 1999. The Ancure endovascular AAA repair system (Guidant Corp., Menlo Park, CA) was approved first, by a margin of a few weeks. This system is a unibody, bifurcated device that is unsupported by a frame but uses hooks and barbs at its proximal and distal attachment sites for aortic and iliac fixation. The system is not available for commercial use in the United States and has been withdrawn from the market.

The AneuRx system, the second endovascular device to receive FDA approval in 1999 for commercial distribution, is based on a modular component design with complete graft support by an external nitinol frame. This system also includes accessory, covered stents of various diameters that can be used selectively to seal endoleaks, to extend the main body of the endograft proximally, or to extend the iliac limbs distally (Figure 10.2).

## Design and development

Dr Thomas J. Fogarty designed the AneuRx stent graft device at Fogarty Engineering in 1993 [5]. The goal was to produce a device that was simple to construct endoluminally and that would eliminate difficult guidewire manipulations. The device was a Dacron graft–based system composed of modular components which was supported throughout its length by a nitinol frame. With modular components of various lengths and diameters, the device could be individualized for the aortic and iliac anatomical variation among patients. The nitinol exoskeleton was incorporated into the design to decrease limb occlusions resulting from extrinsic compression from tortuous or narrowed arterial segments (Figure 10.3).

The original AneuRx device was composed of a thin-walled Dacron graft that was mounted on a nitinol exoskeleton by numerous individual sutures. The nitinol frame was constructed of self-expanding stent rings that were

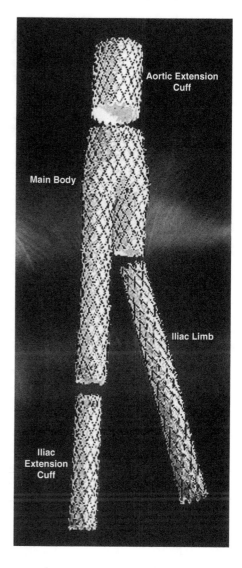

**Figure 10.2** The AneuRx (Medtronic, Inc.) modular, bifurcated endovascular graft with accessory aortic extension cuff and iliac components.

adjacent to one another throughout the length of the graft. The exoskeleton provided columnar support to the graft as well as radial force to achieve apposition of the graft to the aorta for adequate proximal and distal seals. Fixation proximally and distally was maintained by a variable-compression fit (by friction), without the use of hooks or barbs. The main body of the device was supported by a 5-cm stent that was difficult and potentially dangerous to manipulate in tortuous vessels. This stent assembly was modified during clinical trials in 1998, with FDA approval, to replace the stiff 5-cm stent with a series of adjacent 1-cm stents. This modification greatly enhanced the flexibility and maneuverability of the device.

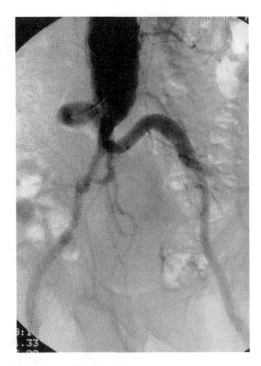

**Figure 10.3** Abdominal aortogram depicting extensive iliac artery tortuosity that may prohibit safe access to the abdominal aorta for endovascular devices.

The development and animal testing of the device was performed by AneuRx, Stanford University Medical Center, and Harbor-UCLA Medical Center. Dr Rodney White implanted the first AneuRx device in the United States at Harbor-UCLA in 1996. The first European deployment was in the Netherlands later that year. The US phase 2 clinical trials for the device began in 1997. After review of the 1-year results of this trial, the FDA panel recommended approval in September 1999.

## Patient selection and graft deployment

Among patients identified with nonruptured AAA who have met the accepted indications for AAA repair, candidates are selected for treatment with the AneuRx stent graft on the basis of the following anatomical criteria: (1) adequate length of infrarenal aortic neck (≥1.0 cm) with minimal angulation, (2) adequate aortic neck diameter (18–26 cm), (3) patent iliac arteries with adequate diameter to accept the delivery catheters (≥6 mm), and (4) limited iliac tortuosity (Figure 10.4).

Unpublished data from our institution suggest that severe aortic neck angulation is associated with a significant increase in perioperative complications

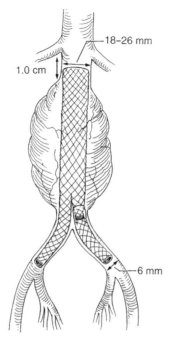

18–26 mm

1.0 cm

6 mm

**Figure 10.4** Anatomical criteria for AneuRx (Medtronic, Inc.) endovascular graft placement.

and an overall poorer outcome [6]. At the Ochsner Clinic in New Orleans, Louisiana, 124 consecutive patients underwent endovascular AAA repair with various devices, including the AneuRx ($n$ = 81), Ancure ($n$ = 9), and Zenith (Cook, Inc., Bloomington, IN) ($n$ = 34) systems. Aortic neck angulation of 60° or more was the only variable associated with a 70% increase in the occurrence of adverse events such as death within 30 days ($P$ < 0.001), conversion to open repair ($P$ < 0.01), aneurysmal expansion ($P$ < 0.01), device migration ($P$ < 0.05), and required secondary procedure ($P$ < 0.001) (Figure 10.5). Similarly, patients with a moderate degree of aortic neck angulation (40–60°) had an intermediate risk (27.8%) of having an adverse event as compared with those with minimal angulation (<40%). These data suggest that the degree of proximal aortic neck angulation significantly affects the overall outcome of endovascular AAA repair. Also, we recommend that in the presence of proximal aortic neck angulation of >60°, endovascular AAA repair should be done only under highly selected circumstances; unless contraindicated, open repair should be considered in patients with a proximal aortic neck angulation of 40–60° (Figure 10.6).

Currently, the AneuRx device is commonly deployed with the use of systemic heparinization and spinal or epidural anesthesia. The femoral arteries are accessed through bilateral femoral cutdown incisions. The device has been deployed percutaneously with the aid of multiple percutaneous closure

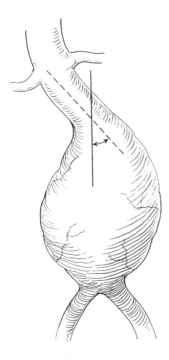

**Figure 10.5** Measurement of aortic neck angulation.

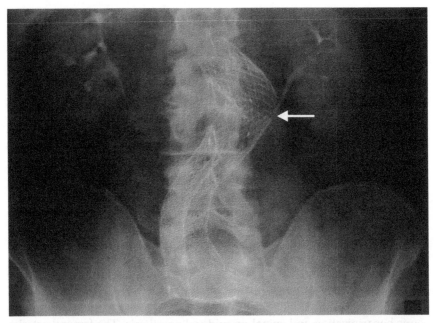

**Figure 10.6** KUB demonstrating inferior migration of the AneuRx (Medtronic, Inc.) main body, which resulted in a delayed endoleak. Arrow indicates migration of main body from aortic cuff extension.

devices used simultaneously, but the overall complication rate of this technique is user dependent [7]. Before deployment of the device, an angiogram is performed with a marker catheter or radiopaque ruler to identify the location of the renal arteries.

The AneuRx device is loaded into 22F (main body) and 16F (contralateral iliac component) deployment sheaths that are inserted into position with femoral arteriotomies. Each sheath is positioned over a 0.035-inch superstiff Amplatz guidewire (Boston Scientific Corp., Natick, MA). The main body and the ipsilateral iliac limb, which are one unit, are deployed initially and then the contralateral iliac limb is deployed within the short contralateral limb (gate) of the main body. The main body of the device is available in 13.5-cm and 16.5-cm lengths. On some occasions, aortic balloon inflations are performed proximally and distally to enhance the apposition of the device to the aortic and iliac wall or to the graft–graft interface. Completion angiography is performed to identify endoleaks (type I or III) that require immediate correction.

After satisfactory stent graft deployment, the femoral arteriotomies are closed by standard vascular surgical technique. Distal lower extremity perfusion should be evaluated before the conclusion of each case.

Endograft surveillance should include abdominal radiography (KUB) with bilateral oblique views as well as an abdominal computed tomographic (CT) scan with and without contrast medium within 30 days of the procedure. Subsequent abdominal CT scans should be performed routinely at 3, 6, and 12 months postoperatively and then annually thereafter. If endoleaks or aneurysmal expansion are noted, further evaluation is essential. In the presence of a type II endoleak, if AAA volume decreases, our policy is to continue careful serial observation. However, AAA expansion that occurs with a known endoleak warrants full, aggressive elucidation, as does significant expansion under any circumstance.

## Early results

The early results of AAA repair using the AneuRx stent graft were published in 1999 in two independent reports of the experiences in the United States and Europe [8,9]. The first published report included data from phase 1 and phase 2 FDA clinical trials that were conducted as multicenter, prospective, nonrandomized investigations comparing open AAA repair and endovascular AAA repair [8]. A total of 250 patients were treated for AAA by open ($n = 60$) or endovascular ($n = 190$) techniques at 12 investigational sites. The AneuRx device was used exclusively in all patients who underwent endovascular repair. The indications for AAA repair and selection of patients for endovascular repair in this study were reported previously [1]. There were no statistical differences between the groups for comorbidities, operative risk (by the ASA [American Society of Anesthesiologists] classification), or AAA size.

Successful stent graft deployment was accomplished in 185 of 190 patients (97%), as compared with 100% procedural success in the open repair group. Among the five procedural failures, severe iliac tortuosity prevented retrograde access to the aorta in four patients; the procedure was aborted for the fifth because the patient had a myocardial infarction on induction of anesthesia. There were no differences between the two groups in anesthesia time or procedure time; however, in the endovascular group there were statistically significant decreases in the volume of blood loss ($P < 0.01$), the number of transfusions ($P < 0.01$), and the duration of hospital stay ($P < 0.01$). There were no conversions to open surgery in the endovascular group. At the time of hospital dismissal, primary technical success for the patients treated with the AneuRx device was 77%, with a 21% rate of endoleaks. There was no significant difference in primary or secondary procedure success between the open and endovascular groups. The reported 6-month graft patency was 98% in the open surgery group and 97% in the endovascular group. At 6-month follow-up, successful AAA exclusion was found in 100% of open repairs and 91% of AAAs treated by endovascular repair. Three patients were identified who had late endoleaks owing to stent graft migration. Each was treated successfully by endovascular placement of AneuRx aortic extension cuff prostheses.

There was no statistical difference in mortality between the open and endovascular groups. No operative mortality was recorded in the open group and five perioperative deaths (2.6%) occurred in the endovascular group, none of which were categorized as device-related. Major morbidity, as defined by the authors, occurred in 23% of the open surgical patients versus 12% of the patients treated with stent graft ($P = 0.03$). The total combined morbidity/mortality rate in the open surgical group (30%) was not significantly different from that in the endovascular group (19%). There were no AAA ruptures in either group of patients. The data from this initial report on the AneuRx device facilitated subsequent clinical trials that ultimately led to FDA approval of the device.

The second report published in 1999 was a prospective study aimed at evaluating the safety and efficacy of the AneuRx device at 1-year follow-up [9]. With others, Dr R.P. Tutein Nolthenius at St Antonius Hospital in the Netherlands reported on a series of 104 patients with AAA treated with the AneuRx device between December 1996 and November 1997 at four centers in Europe. The authors reported successful AneuRx stent graft deployment in 102 of 104 patients (98%). Of the two patients who underwent immediate conversion to open AAA repair, one had severe iliac tortuosity and the other had unsuccessful positioning of the contralateral limb within the main body of the device. No device-related failures were reported in this series. There were two deaths in the perioperative period which were not felt to be device-related; both patients had severe comorbidities and were at increased risk of perioperative mortality (ASA class IV). A total of 38 aortic extension cuffs were placed in 34 patients to achieve complete AAA exclusion. Seven of these were placed at the proximal aortic attachment site because of type I endoleaks. There were no technical failures among the patients receiving the stent graft.

All patients were accounted for in follow-up (range, 12–24 months). There was no evidence of stent graft migration or limb occlusion owing to kinking of the endograft. One graft limb occlusion was identified at 6 months postoperatively. The cause of this limb occlusion was believed to be incomplete expansion of the device across an iliac stenosis. This was treated successfully by thrombolysis and percutaneous transluminal angioplasty. At 12-month follow-up, there were four persistent endoleaks and no sign of AAA expansion. Therefore, continued surveillance was recommended.

This series demonstrated consistent success for the procedure in a select group of AAA patients as well as several benefits of the endovascular technique of AAA repair. The authors cited a short operative time, decreased length of stay overall and in intensive care units, and a relatively rapid recovery as compared with open AAA repair historical controls [10]. They also wisely recommended the need for randomized, prospective investigations comparing open repair and endovascular AAA repair.

## AneuRx FDA clinical trials: 4-year results

Zarins et al. [11] reported the cumulative data collected from FDA clinical trials (phases 1, 2, and 3) of the AneuRx device in February 2001. The goal of this review was to determine the outcome of endovascular AAA repair using the AneuRx device on an intent-to-treat basis. The primary end points of this study were AAA rupture, death from AAA rupture, death from any cause, conversion to open AAA repair, and secondary procedures due to endoleaks, occlusions, or migration. These data were collected from a cohort of a total of 1192 patients who participated in the endovascular treatment arm of the clinical trials from June 1996 through November 1999, with a mean ($\pm$ SD) follow-up of 73.4 $\pm$ 8.0 months. This included 87 patients who were treated on a compassionate-use basis in phases 2 and 3.

The characteristics of the 1192 patients were similar to those of the individual trials, with 1058 men (89%) and 134 women (11%) who had a mean age of 73.4 years (range, 45–96 years). The comorbidities and operative risk factors were characteristic of any large group of patients with aneurysms. Most of the patients (92%) were classified in ASA risk category III or IV. The mean dimensions of the AAAs were as follows: diameter, 5.6 cm; aortic neck length, 27.3 mm; and aortic neck diameter, 22.3 mm.

### Rupture and mortality

The most important primary end points of this comprehensive analysis were the rate of rupture and survival after endovascular repair. A total of 10 AAA ruptures (0.8%) were reported among the 1192 patients who received the AneuRx device in the United States as of June 2000. Two of the ruptures occurred as a result of the implantation procedure. Each patient was hemodynamically unstable immediately after the procedure. After resuscitation, abdominal CT scans showed large retroperitoneal hematomas in both cases. Each patient was returned to the operating room and underwent successful open AAA repair: one with an aortobifemoral reconstruction and the other with an aortobiiliac reconstruction. In both cases, aortic perforations were found at the time of repair. The other eight AAA ruptures were delayed, occurring in an average of 17 months (range, 3 weeks to 26 months) postoperatively. Successful open AAA repair was performed in five of these patients, two died during the perioperative period, and one died after refusing operative intervention. In 6 of the 10 patients, no evidence of endoleak or AAA enlargement was identified. Four of the ruptures resulted from a failure of proximal fixation, presumably owing to highly angulated aortic necks. The other two ruptures resulted from separation of the modular components at the interface of the iliac limb and main body of the device. Endovascular placement of aortic extension cuffs potentially could have been used to repair each of these device failures. Similarly, the other two patients who experienced AAA rupture had type I distal endoleaks amenable to endovascular correction, but each refused treatment.

The overall mortality rate of the 1192 patients who received the AneuRx device was 10%. A total of 119 patients died within 4 years after the initial device was implanted. The reported 30-day mortality was 2% (23 of 1192 patients). Aside from the 10 AAA ruptures described previously, the other patient deaths were from cardiac disease in 49 patients, cancer in 20, pulmonary disease in 19, renal disease in 7, multisystem organ failure in 5, gastrointestinal tract disease in 4, stroke in 3, pulmonary embolism in 1, and mesenteric ischemia in 1. For four patients, the cause of death was not determined. The overall survival by Kaplan-Meier life table analysis was 93% at 1 year, 88% at 2 years, and 86% at 3 years.

## Endoleak

The incidence of endoleaks among patients treated with the AneuRx stent graft was evaluated in 398 of the 425 patients who participated in the endovascular treatment arm of the phase 2 clinical trial [12]. Abdominal CT scans, with and without contrast medium enhancement, were performed within 1 week after device implantation for 98% of the patients. Endoleaks were identified at each investigational site in 152 of the 398 patients (38%). After review of the CT scans at the core laboratory, 175 patients (44%) were identified as having an endoleak in the perioperative period. The total endoleak rate reported by the centers was 13% at 1 month, 16% at 6 months, and 13% at 12 months. The results of the core laboratory analysis indicated an endoleak rate of 27% at 6 months and 20% at 1 year; 54 patients (31%) had type I endoleaks, 70 (40%) had type II endoleaks, and 51 (29%) had endoleaks of undetermined type.

During the period from 2 weeks to 16 months postimplantation, 15 patients received additional endovascular treatment. Nine of the 15 patients had an endoleak that was identified before dismissal; six had endoleaks that developed after dismissal or were not evident on the initial imaging. Proximal aortic extension cuffs were used in eight patients, distal extension cuffs in five, and proximal and distal extension cuffs in two. The endoleaks were successfully eliminated in nine patients; the leak persisted in the other six patients.

The actual predictive value of an endoleak after endovascular AAA repair is unclear. Although it would seem logical that an endoleak is an ominous sign, by Kaplan-Meier life table analysis, there was no difference in mortality between patients with a known endoleak (5%) seen on predischarge CT scan and the patients with no endoleak (5%) at 1 month. Similarly, at 1-month follow-up no statistically significant differences were found for aneurysmal expansion, stent graft migration, or rupture between patients with and without endoleaks. Overall, the survival after endovascular AAA repair with the AneuRx device in this phase 2 trial was 96% by life table analysis at 12 months and was independent of endoleak status.

## Stent graft migration

One of the primary criticisms of endovascular AAA repair involves the effect of the morphologic changes to the aneurysm sac and aortic neck that occur over time. Aortic neck enlargement has been demonstrated in patients after open as well as endovascular AAA repair [13]. This aortic expansion may result in delayed type I proximal endoleaks or stent graft migration, or both, and ultimately pressurization of the AAA and subsequent rupture. Deliberate oversizing of the proximal device by up to 20% has become widely accepted to combat the problem of aortic neck enlargement. Also, manufacturers have engineered various structural innovations to achieve proximal device fixation. The AneuRx device uses friction and radial compression force from its self-expanding stent exoskeleton to secure the proximal attachment site. Undoubtedly, the actual incidence of stent graft migration is underreported because it is easily missed and, when noted, corrected by endovascular placement of proximal aortic extension cuffs.

In the initial published report comparing AneuRx endovascular AAA repair with open repair, migration of the device was identified in 3 of 190 patients (1.6%) at 1-year follow-up, resulting in a proximal endoleak in two cases and a type III endoleak in the third [8]. The proximal migrations were 1 cm or less and were felt to be the result of low initial deployment of the stent graft. This would result in an inadequate area of contact between the device and the aortic neck, reducing the friction and radial force applied by the exoskeleton. The third stent graft migration resulted in an endoleak between the contralateral iliac limb and the bifurcated main body of the device. Again, this problem was believed to be the result of an error in the initial implantation procedure, with inadequate overlap of the contralateral limb within the gate of the main body in association with a tortuous iliac artery. In each case, the endoleak was successfully treated with endovascular deployment of proximal aortic or iliac extension cuffs.

Because stent graft migration may occur over an extended period, CT scans and abdominal radiographs need to be evaluated over extended periods of follow-up. In our experience, migration has led to delayed endoleaks without obvious changes on CT scans. Because the risk of migration continues over time, continued surveillance is in order. The true causes of migration are not fully elucidated, and it is possible that elongation of the aorta in concert with proximal or distal dilation may be responsible for this problem.

## Comparison with open repair

In general, endovascular AAA repair has been shown to decrease the morbidity, blood loss, length of hospital stay, and time to return to normal level of activity [1,14]. The results of the phase 2 clinical trial of the AneuRx device showed no significant difference in survival at 1 year between patients treated with the endovascular device and those treated with open surgical repair [8]. With the relatively recent development of endovascular AAA repair, the authors feel it would be premature to make any meaningful comparisons in terms of survival between the open and endovascular surgical techniques. The decrease in mortality in the endovascular group that was expected by some has yet to be realized. Similarly, no study has demonstrated a decrease in combined morbidity/mortality. These findings are especially significant because the largest patient groups studied to date in the United States have included select patients who would not be classified at increased risk for open surgical AAA repair. It seems intuitive, however, that some selection of higher risk patients is occurring.

## Future developments

Advancements in endovascular technology seem to occur daily. Device designers are planning improvements to make the next generation of devices safer, easier to deploy, more adaptable to anatomical complexities, and more effective. The anticipated modifications to the AneuRx device include a tapered nose cone for improved delivery through tortuous iliac arteries and an integrated deployment system. This new system would eliminate the reel device currently in use. Information about further improvements in the AneuRx device has not yet become publicly available.

One interesting application of the AneuRx technology has been the use of the aortic extension cuffs in a stacked configuration to create a tube endograft for the exclusion of saccular AAA (Figure 10.7) [15]. In this series, five patients underwent successful endovascular repair of saccular infrarenal AAA with only AneuRx aortic cuffs. Each patient was found to have asymptomatic saccular AAA with ample normal native aorta proximally and distally to the AAA. Cuffs of appropriate diameter were deployed sequentially with an overlap of at least 1.5 cm to fashion a tube endograft that excluded the saccular aneurysm. Each AAA was completely excluded with no sign of endoleak

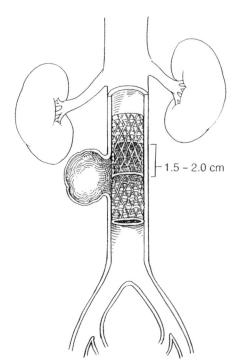

1.5 – 2.0 cm

**Figure 10.7** AneuRx (Medtronic, Inc.)
aortic extension cuffs deployed in a stacked
configuration.

or device migration at 12-month follow-up. Owing to the uncertain natural
history of saccular AAA, the appropriate timing of repair is accordingly not
well defined. This application of the AneuRx components has proved to be a
valuable endovascular technique for treating this type of aneurysm, which
may have otherwise gone untreated if the alternative were open aortic reconstruction for a relatively small, asymptomatic AAA.

## Summary

The AneuRx endovascular AAA repair system has been shown to be an effective therapy for prevention of AAA rupture in US clinical trials as well as in
the worldwide experience. The device has been shown to be 99.5% effective
in patients treated and followed up for 4 years. Although no long-term results
are available beyond 4 years, the results to date are encouraging. In the current
state of development, it is uncertain whether endovascular AAA repair will
replace open surgical AAA repair or simply satisfy a need for a less invasive
treatment option in unfit surgical patients. The ultimate fate of this technology, we hope, will be decided by the time-honored standards of experience
and well-designed investigational studies.

# References

1 May J, White GH, Yu W *et al.* Concurrent comparison of endoluminal versus open repair in the treatment of abdominal aortic aneurysms: analysis of 303 patients by life table method. *J Vasc Surg* 1998; **27**: 213–20.

2 Moore WS, Kashyap VS, Vescera CL, Quinones-Baldrich WJ. Abdominal aortic aneurysm: a 6-year comparison of endovascular versus transabdominal repair. *Ann Surg* 1999; **230**: 298–306.

3 Dubost C, Allary M, Oeconomos N. Resection of an aneurysm of the abdominal aorta; reestablishment of continuity by preserved human arterial graft, with results after 5 months. *Arch Surg* 1952; **64**: 405–8.

4 Parodi JC, Palmaz JC, Barone HD. Transfemoral intraluminal graft implantation for abdominal aortic aneurysms. *Ann Vasc Surg* 1991; **5**: 491–9.

5 Allen RC, Zarins CK, Fogarty TJ. The Medtronic-AneuRx modular bifurcated graft. In: Yao JST, Pearce WH, eds. *Techniques in Vascular and Endovascular Surgery.* Stamford, CT: Appelton & Lange, 1998: 401–9.

6 Sternbergh WC III, Carter G, York JW, Yoselevitz M, Money SR. Aortic neck angulation predicts adverse outcome with endovascular abdominal aortic aneurysm repair. *J Vasc Surg* 2002; **35**: 482–6.

7 Traul DK, Clair DG, Gray B, O'Hara PJ, Ouriel K. Percutaneous endovascular repair of infrarenal abdominal aortic aneurysms: a feasibility study. *J Vasc Surg* 2000; **32**: 770–6.

8 Zarins CK, White RA, Schwarten D *et al.* AneuRx stent graft versus open surgical repair of abdominal aortic aneurysms: multicenter prospective clinical trial. *J Vasc Surg* 1999; **29**: 292–305.

9 Tutein Nolthenius RP, vd Berg JC, Biasi GM *et al.* Endoluminal repair of infrarenal abdominal aortic aneurysms using a modular stent-graft: one-year clinical results from a European multicentre trial. *Cardiovasc Surg* 1999; **7**: 503–7.

10 White GH, May J, McGahan T *et al.* Historic control comparison of outcome for matched groups of patients undergoing endoluminal versus open repair of abdominal aortic aneurysms. *J Vasc Surg* 1996; **23**: 201–11.

11 Zarins CK, White RA, Moll FL *et al.* The AneuRx stent graft: four-year results and world-wide experience 2000. *J Vasc Surg* 2001; **33**(Suppl): S135–45. Erratum in: *J Vasc Surg* 2001; **33**: 1318.

12 Zarins CK, White RA, Hodgson KJ, Schwarten D, Fogarty TJ. Endoleak as a predictor of outcome after endovascular aneurysm repair: AneuRx multicenter clinical trial. *J Vasc Surg* 2000; **32**: 90–107.

13 Matsumura JS, Chaikof EL. Anatomic changes after endovascular grafting for aneurysmal disease. *Semin Vasc Surg* 1999; **12**: 192–8.

14 Brewster DC, Geller SC, Kaufman JA *et al.* Initial experience with endovascular aneurysm repair: comparison of early results with outcome of conventional open repair. *J Vasc Surg* 1998; **27**: 992–1003.

15 York JW, Sternbergh WC III, Lepore MR, Money SR. Endovascular exclusion of saccular abdominal aortic aneurysms using "stacked" AneuRx aortic cuffs. Retrieved December 31, 2003 from the World Wide Web: http://www.pvss.org/Wabs2001/abstracts01-6.pdf.

# CHAPTER 11

# Excluder bifurcated endoprosthesis system

Eric T. Choi, MD, Gregorio A. Sicard, MD

## Introduction

The Excluder bifurcated endoprosthesis (W.L. Gore and Associates, Inc., Flagstaff, AZ) is an endovascular device that is undergoing clinical investigation to test its efficacy in the treatment of abdominal aortic aneurysms (AAAs). Several studies have been conducted since it received US Food and Drug Administration (FDA) approval for the investigational device exemption in 1997. In this chapter, we present the technical and short-term results with this endograft from the US phase 1 and phase 2 trials, our institutional experience, and an international multicenter registry, EUROSTAR (European Collaborators on Stent-Graft Techniques for Abdominal Aortic Aneurysm Repair). The US phase 2 trial has been completed and the 12- and 24-month data were reviewed by the FDA Circulatory Devices Panel in September 2002, leading to conditional approval of the Excluder device. In November 2002, full FDA approval for commercial use was granted.

## Description of the device

The Excluder device is manufactured for the treatment of infrarenal AAAs. It is a modular bifurcated endograft composed of a nitinol stent exoskeleton and a graft cover made of polytetrafluoroethylene spanning the length of the stent without suture holes (Figure 11.1). The proximal attachment system has eight pairs of anchors to provide increased proximal fixation to counteract the radial force of the nitinol stent. The main advantage of the Excluder endograft over other commercially available devices (e.g., the AneuRx stent graft [Medtronic, Inc., Minneapolis, MN] and the Ancure stent graft [Guidant Corp., Menlo Park, CA]) is the low profile of the main device and contralateral limb. This advantage has been demonstrated by the 100% technical success achieved with this device, which is clearly superior to the success rates of the other commercially available devices.

The components used in the US phase 1 and phase 2 FDA trials were available in several aortic and iliac diameters and lengths. Each trunk component has a contralateral limb attachment site, which accommodates different iliac diameters and lengths and allows different iliac diameters to be used with

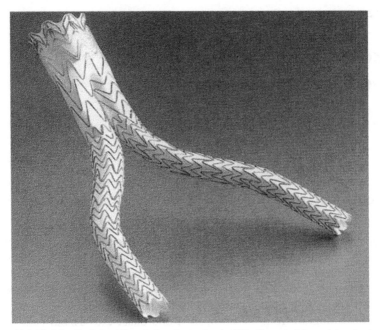

**Figure 11.1** Modular Excluder bifurcated endoprosthesis (W.L. Gore and Associates, Inc.).

any aortic diameter. This contrasts with the current standard open aortic grafts or other FDA-approved endovascular devices (e.g., the Ancure and AneuRx devices), which are available with iliac limbs that have equal diameters that are approximately one-half the size of the aortic diameter. Components for aortic and iliac extension are also available with the Excluder and were used by the investigators in the US and European trials.

The Excluder endoprosthesis has a flexible delivery system to decrease the risk of arterial injury during insertion. An 18F sheath is used to introduce the trunk, and a 12F sheath is used to introduce the contralateral limb components (Figure 11.2). Radiopaque markers are present along the length of every component for fluoroscopic visualization. After the deployment system is positioned, the components are rapidly deployed by a pull-cord mechanism with minimal foreshortening on release (Figure 11.3).

## Inclusion criteria

The available aortic diameters of the main body of the Excluder endoprosthesis are 23, 26, and 28.5 mm; the available diameters of the distal ipsilateral limb are 12 and 14.5 mm; and the available lengths of the distal ipsilateral limb are 14, 16, and 18 cm. The available diameters of the distal contralateral limb are 12 and 14 mm, and the available lengths are 10, 12, and 14 cm. Oversizing

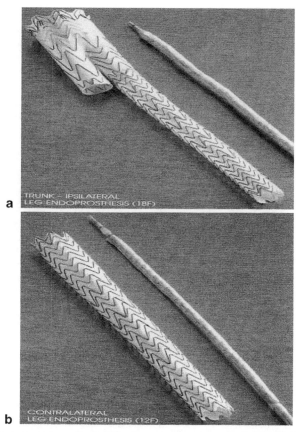

**Figure 11.2** Excluder endoprosthesis (W.L. Gore and Associates, Inc.). (a) Main body (trunk and ipsilateral limb) with undeployed contralateral limb. (b) Deployed contralateral limb.

by 10–20% is recommended for the aortic site and for the iliac attachment sites. The anatomical indications for use of the Excluder in the treatment of AAA are as follows: (1) aortic neck diameter between 19 and 26.5 mm, (2) common iliac artery diameter between 10 and 13.5 mm, (3) external iliac artery diameter between 8 and 13.5 mm (if the external iliac artery is used), (4) proximal aortic neck angulation of no more than 60°, (5) proximal aortic neck length of 15 mm or more, and (6) common iliac artery sealing length of 10 mm or more.

## FDA Phase 1 trial

For the first US trial, 29 subjects were enrolled in three centers (27 men [93%] and two women [7%]; mean age, 76 years; range, 59–91 years) from January 1998 through October 1998, as previously reported [1]. The mean maximal

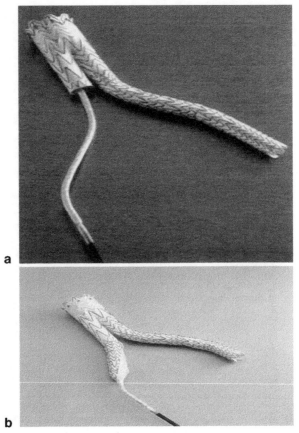

**Figure 11.3** Excluder endoprosthesis (W.L. Gore and Associates, Inc.). (a) *In vitro* cannulation of contralateral limb cage. (b) Deployment of contralateral limb.

aneurysm diameter was 5.7 cm (range, 4.5–9.0 cm), and the aneurysm classification by the Society for Vascular Surgery/International Society for Cardiovascular Surgery reporting standards [2] was I for 25 subjects (86%), II for three subjects (10%), and III for one subject (3%). The New York Heart Association classification was I for 22 subjects (76%), II for five subjects (17%), and III for two subjects (7%); none were in class IV.

## Procedure

The Excluder AAA procedure was performed with general, epidural or spinal, or local anesthesia and involved bilateral groin incisions for exposure of the common femoral arteries. Adjunctive brachial artery catheterization was used according to the surgeon's discretion. Fixed or mobile fluoroscopy imaging and power-injector angiography were used to guide the placement of the stent graft. Aorto-uni-iliac implantations required exclusion of the contralateral iliac artery by surgical ligation or coil embolization (or a combination of the two) and by crossover femorofemoral bypass grafting.

Deployment success was defined as the ability to deliver the stent graft into position as intended. Technical success was defined as successful deployment without endoleak at the time of the initial procedure. Adverse events were defined as any complication that required additional procedures or prolonged hospitalization, or both (e.g., arterial rupture or dissection, renal dysfunction, lower extremity ischemia, significant cardiac or respiratory complications, and conversion to open AAA repair).

## Follow-up evaluation

Patients underwent abdominal radiography and spiral computed tomography (with or without contrast enhancement) before hospital dismissal to evaluate device placement, graft patency, aneurysm size, renal artery patency, and presence or absence of endoleak. These studies were reviewed locally at each site and at an independent core laboratory facility. After hospital dismissal, the patients were evaluated at 1 month, 6 months, 1 year, and yearly thereafter.

## Results

The deployment and technical successes were 100%. There were no immediate conversions. No postoperative or in-hospital deaths occurred. Thirteen patients had 21 complications (Table 11.1). Because adverse events were the primary focus of this study, these complications were followed closely and were presented in detail by Matsumura and colleagues [1]. Briefly, many complications were related to the procedure and reflected the significant risks associated with these vascular procedures. Two patients had iliac artery dissections that were treated endoluminally or resolved spontaneously on follow-up. One patient experienced a reaction to contrast medium. In two patients, ipsilateral groin wound lymph leak developed, which spontaneously resolved. One had an arteriovenous fistula that was noted in the groin after dismissal. In one patient, an endograft infection was detected 1 month after stent graft placement when the patient presented with fever and back pain. Blood cultures were positive for *Staphylococcus aureus*, and aspirate samples of perigraft fluid also showed *S. aureus*. The patient was treated with antibiotics, extra-anatomic bypass, and staged explantation of the endoprosthesis.

## Endoleaks

The investigators reported an endoleak rate after dismissal of 39% at 3 months, 23% at 6 months, and 16% at 12 months. Most patients (60%) had type II endoleaks. Three patients had a proximal attachment site endoleak, two of which resolved spontaneously and one of which persisted in a patient with an aneurysm that had a short, angled proximal neck. The aneurysm in

**Table 11.1** Number of adverse events in 13 patients in the US phase 1 trial of the excluder bifurcated endoprosthesis (W.L. Gore and Associates, Inc.).

| Adverse event | At dismissal* | After dismissal,* months | | |
|---|---|---|---|---|
| | | 3 | 6 | 12 |
| Death | – | – | – | – |
| Myocardial infarction | – | – | – | – |
| Arrhythmia | – | – | 1 | – |
| Angina | – | 1 | – | – |
| Stroke | – | – | – | – |
| Transient ischemic attack | – | – | – | 1 |
| Endograft infection | – | 1 | – | – |
| Renal thrombosis | – | 1 | – | – |
| Acute renal failure | 1 | – | – | – |
| Procedural blood loss | 1 | – | – | – |
| Hematoma | 1 | – | – | – |
| Seroma/lymphocele | 1 | 3 | – | – |
| Arteriovenous fistula | 1 | – | – | – |
| Iliac artery dissection | 1 | 1 | – | – |
| Deep venous thrombosis | – | 1 | – | – |
| Buttock/thigh claudication | 1 | 2 | – | – |
| Testicular pain | – | – | 1 | – |
| Contrast medium reaction | – | – | 1 | – |

*Dash indicates no adverse event.
(Reprinted from Matsumura JS, Katzen BT, Hollier LH, Dake MD, Update on the bifurcated EXCLUDER endoprosthesis: phase I results, *J Vasc Surg* 2001; **33** (Suppl): S150–3, Copyright 2001, with permission from The Society for Vascular Surgery and The American Association for Vascular Surgery [1].)

this patient has not increased in size, and she is not a candidate for treatment with an aortic cuff because of severe angulation. She has refused conversion to open AAA repair. At 12 months, there were no aneurysmal ruptures, limb thromboses, endograft migrations, or aneurysm-related deaths.

## FDA phase 2 trial (the Pivotal Excluder study)

The Pivotal Excluder study was conducted from December 28, 1998, through January 26, 2000, at 19 investigational US centers. Results from this endovascular treatment arm, which enrolled 235 patients treated with the Excluder endograft, were compared with results from 99 control patients treated with open AAA repair. The total supravalvular aortic stenosis risk factor score was 4 for both groups. The technical success for the Excluder group was 100%. Statistically significant differences between the two groups, in favor of the Excluder-treated patients, were observed in mean procedure time ($P < 0.0001$), need for homologous blood ($P < 0.0001$), mean length of stay in the intensive

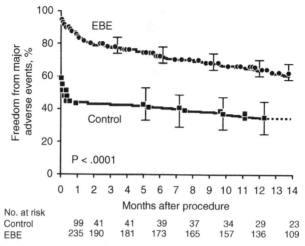

**Figure 11.4** Freedom from first adverse events in phase 2 trial comparing the group receiving the Excluder bifurcated endoprosthesis (EBE) (W.L. Gore and Associates, Inc.) with the control group that underwent open surgical repair in the treatment of abdominal aortic aneurysms. (Data from W.L. Gore and Associates, Inc., pers. comm., 2004.)

care unit ($P < 0.0001$), mean length of hospital stay ($P < 0.0001$), time to ambulation ($P < 0.0001$), and return to normal activities ($P = 0.002$).

At 1, 6, and 12 months, freedom from first adverse events in the Excluder group was statistically higher (86%, 74%, and 62%, respectively) than in the open repair group (43%, 43%, and 35%, respectively) (Figure 11.4). Patient survival at 12 and 24 months was similar for both groups. No aneurysmal rupture or aneurysm-related deaths have occurred. Reinterventions have been required in 7% of the patients in the first year and 7% in the second year of follow-up. Three patients required open conversion and one patient required an iliorenal bypass to revascularize an occlusion of a renal artery. Most reinterventions (87%) were performed endoluminally.

## Washington University Medical Center experience

From March 1999 through February 2001, as part of the FDA phase 2 trial, 33 patients underwent elective endoluminal AAA repair with the Excluder endoprosthesis at Washington University Medical Center, St Louis, Missouri. Spinal anesthesia was used in 85% of the procedures and general anesthesia in 15%. The mean age of the patients was 74.6 years (range, 50–92 years); 24 patients (73%) were men and nine (27%) were women. The mean aortic diameter was 5.5 cm. The technical success was 100%, with a mean operating room time of 136 min. Three patients had postoperative complications: two had incisional groin lymphoceles that required surgical treatment, which was successful, and one had a ventricular arrhythmia that required intravenous antiarrhythmic therapy. The mean length of hospital stay was 1.5 days.

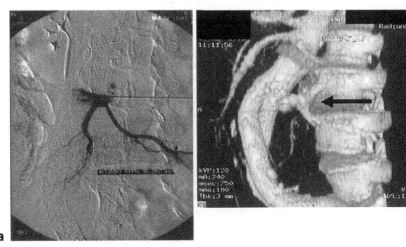

**Figure 11.5** (a) Translumbar puncture for glue embolization in a persistent type II endoleak associated with aneurysmal growth. (b) Three-dimensional reconstruction 6 months after glue embolization of a type II endoleak. Note glue cast (arrow).

During a mean follow-up of 24.5 months after Excluder implantation, five patients died, but there were no aneurysm-related deaths: two died of myocardial infarction (at 2 and 5 months) and three died of malignancy (at 16, 17, and 32 months). In our experience, only one patient has required open conversion at 20 months after implantation because of endotension (no endoleak apparent on contrast computed tomography or arteriography), with aneurysm sac growth from 6.5 to 7.8 cm. In one patient, a new type II endoleak developed at 6 months, and at 12 months the aneurysm sac had grown 8 mm, requiring translumbar embolization with glue, which was successful (Figure 11.5).

## European EUROSTAR trial

The EUROSTAR trial collected data on the use of the Excluder device from January 1998 through July 2001 from 33 centers throughout Europe. We report the 24-month follow-up results (W.L. Gore and Associates, Inc., personal communication, 2004). Among the 234 patients treated with the Excluder endograft, the mean age was 71 years, (range, 50–87 years) and the mean maximal aneurysm diameter was 5.6 cm (range, 3.0–9.4 cm).

Preoperatively, cardiac problems were recorded most frequently. Among the 234 patients, 23% were severely obese, 27% had had a laparotomy, 17% were unfit for an open procedure, and 2% were unfit for general anesthesia. Computed tomography combined with digital subtraction angiography was the preoperative assessment of choice in the majority of the centers.

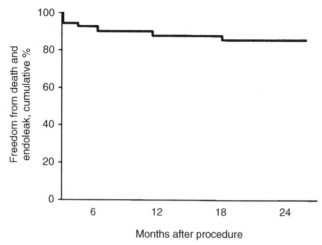

**Figure 11.6** Excluder (W.L. Gore and Associates, Inc.) EUROSTAR (European Collaborators on Stent-Graft Techniques for Abdominal Aortic Aneurysm Repair) data for freedom from death and endoleak at 24 months. (Data from W.L. Gore and Associates, Inc., pers. comm., 2004.)

## Follow-up evaluation

Patients underwent abdominal radiography and spiral computed tomography (with or without contrast enhancement) before hospital dismissal to evaluate device placement, graft patency, aneurysm size, renal artery patency, and presence or absence of endoleak. These studies were reviewed locally at each site and at an independent core laboratory facility. After hospital dismissal, the patients were evaluated at 1, 3, 6, 12, and 18 months, and yearly thereafter.

## Results

The Excluder bifurcated endoprosthesis was used in 234 patients, with one or more limb extensions needed in 18% of the cases. The most frequently used device sizes were a length of 160 mm and a limb diameter of 14 mm.

Technical success was achieved in 100% of the patients. Device-related complications occurred in 12 of 234 cases (5%). In four patients the delivery sheath could not be advanced, and in four the device migrated during deployment.

In the first 6 months of follow-up, no graft migration, stenosis, or thrombosis occurred. At 1-year follow-up, one patient had aneurysmal rupture and one patient had graft thrombosis. Unfortunately, the EUROSTAR authors do not know the circumstances surrounding the ruptured aneurysm. Freedom from death and endoleak was seen in 88% of the patients (Figure 11.6).

## Discussion

US phase 1 and 2 trials, as well as the EUROSTAR trial, have conclusively demonstrated the overall safety and short- and mid-term efficacy of the

Excluder device in the treatment of infrarenal AAA. These three trials have demonstrated that the incidence and severity of adverse events with the use of the Excluder device are comparable to published data for patients who underwent endovascular repair with other devices [3,4]. In the US trials, no deaths or ruptures occurred. Furthermore, the low profile of this endograft allowed a 100% procedural technical success, something not reported with the other commercially available devices. In the EUROSTAR trial, one death occurred from rupture after implantation. It is certain that with more implantations and longer surveillance periods, the risk of rupture per year of implantation will be better defined for this device. Because a primary objective of all treatment methods offered for AAA is avoidance of rupture, lifelong surveillance of endovascular treatment of this condition is imperative. It is encouraging that the Excluder design is not associated with more complications and is associated with a much higher technical success rate than other commercially available endografts. The case of the graft infection in the US phase 1 trial seems to have been an isolated incident.

These Excluder trials reported no greater incidence of technical failures, such as an inability to complete the procedure or limb occlusion. In addition, there was no greater incidence of migration detected with the Excluder than with the FDA-approved endovascular devices [5–8]. With the 18F (for the ipsilateral approach) and the 12F (for the contralateral approach) delivery systems, more patients may be candidates for endovascular treatment of infrarenal AAA, particularly women who have smaller access arteries.

Zarins and colleagues [9] demonstrated that individual investigators underreport sequelae, especially endoleaks, more often than core laboratory investigators. The US phase 2 trial specifically addresses these concerns pertaining to endoleaks and other complications. As far as we know, the endoleak rates in the US phase 1 and phase 2 trials and in the EUROSTAR trial are remarkably similar to those reported with other devices [5–8], both at dismissal and at 12-month follow-up. The usual predominance of type II endoleaks in these studies and others suggests that this type of endoleak will be a universal phenomenon until newer technology is developed. Only long-term evaluation of untreated type II endoleaks (especially if no aneurysm sac growth occurs) will show their clinical significance after AAA endovascular repair.

Despite ongoing doubt and recent concerns surrounding clinical efficacy and durability, endovascular repair of infrarenal AAA is by far the most exciting development in vascular surgery in the past decade. All clinical investigators recognize the somewhat unfinished nature of this endovascular technology that, by all accounts, is still in its infancy. Future developments will most likely address the major unresolved issues, mainly deliverability to the aortic lumen, reliable fixation in challenging proximal necks, and, foremost, the ability to adjust to evolving morphologic changes (as the excluded aneurysm shrinks) without disconnections, dislocations, or migration. Available information is inconclusive on the occurrence of endoleaks and the potential for late aneurysmal rupture after endovascular repair.

In summary, the modular Excluder bifurcated endoprosthesis provides a lower profile and greater flexibility than other endografts. Excellent results from FDA phase 1 and phase 2 trials, as well as data from the EUROSTAR registry, establish the Excluder as a new commercially available endograft that will be an addition to the endoluminal treatment of AAAs.

## References

1 Matsumura JS, Katzen BT, Hollier LH, Dake MD. Update on the bifurcated EXCLUDER endoprosthesis: phase I results. *J Vasc Surg* 2001; **33**(Suppl): S150–3.
2 Ahn SS, Rutherford RB, Johnston KW *et al.*, for the Ad Hoc Committee for Standardized Reporting Practices in Vascular Surgery of The Society for Vascular Surgery/International Society for Cardiovascular Surgery. Reporting standards for infrarenal endovascular abdominal aortic aneurysm repair. *J Vasc Surg* 1997; **25**: 405–10.
3 Moore WS, Brewster DC, Bernhard VM. Aorto-uni-iliac endograft for complex aortoiliac aneurysms compared with tube/bifurcation endografts: results of the EVT/Guidant trials. *J Vasc Surg* 2001; **33**(Suppl): S11–20.
4 Holzenbein TJ, Kretschmer G, Thurnher S *et al.* Midterm durability of abdominal aortic aneurysm endograft repair: a word of caution. *J Vasc Surg* 2001; **33**(Suppl): S46–54.
5 Greenberg RK, Lawrence-Brown M, Bhandari G *et al.* An update of the Zenith endovascular graft for abdominal aortic aneurysms: initial implantation and mid-term follow-up data. *J Vasc Surg* 2001; **33**(Suppl): S157–64.
6 Criado FJ, Wilson EP, Fairman RM, Abul-Khoudoud O, Wellons E. Update on the Talent aortic stent-graft: a preliminary report from United States phase I and II trials. *J Vasc Surg* 2001; **33**(Suppl): S146–9.
7 Zarins CK, White RA, Moll FL *et al.* The AneuRx stent graft: four-year results and worldwide experience 2000. *J Vasc Surg* 2001; **33**(Suppl): S135–45. Published erratum in *J Vasc Surg* 2001; **33**: 1318.
8 Harris PL, Vallabhaneni SR, Desgranges P *et al.*, for the EUROSTAR Collaborators. Incidence and risk factors of late rupture, conversion, and death after endovascular repair of infrarenal aortic aneurysms: the EUROSTAR experience. *J Vasc Surg* 2000; **32**: 739–49.
9 Zarins CK, White RA, Hodgson KJ, Schwarten D, Fogarty TJ. Endoleak as a predictor of outcome after endovascular aneurysm repair: AneuRx multicenter clinical trial. *J Vasc Surg* 2000; **32**: 90–107.

# CHAPTER 12

# Zenith AAA endovascular graft

Beate Neuhauser, MD, W. Andrew Oldenburg, MD, Albert G. Hakaim, MD

## History of the device

The Zenith abdominal aortic aneurysm (AAA) endovascular graft (Cook, Inc., Bloomington, IN) was initially developed and tested at the Royal Perth Hospital in Australia. Guidelines were derived from clinical experience and intuition and from the mechanical and physical principles for endoluminal devices described previously by Stanley et al. [1] after they started their endovascular aortic aneurysm repair program in 1993. The Zenith two-piece aortoiliac modular bifurcated graft formed the initial basic unit for endovascular repair. Ultimately, three-piece units have replaced the two-piece device to provide more flexibility for length and sizing (Figure 12.1).

## Description of the device

The Zenith device is a supported, bifurcated, modular, self-expandable endograft that has multiple stainless steel modified Gianturco Z stents (Cook, Inc.) placed as an exoskeleton, with proximal and distal bare stents placed at a 3-mm stagger. The delivery system, which is inserted into the femoral artery, consists of specialized catheters and guidewires with radiopaque markers for accurate orientation and placement of the device. The bifurcated graft is a three-piece modular unit offering more flexibility in the length and sizing of both limbs than other devices (Figure 12.1). The diameter of the main body ranges from 22 to 32 mm, and the length ranges from 104 to 162 mm; the delivery system uses 18–20F introducers [2]. The proximal end of the main body has a 20-mm-long section of uncovered stent with barbs at the apexes, allowing safe transrenal placement and aortic fixation. Compared with other aortic stent grafts, the main body has a longer aortic component to facilitate cannulation of the contralateral limb. The iliac limb may be flared at the end to form a safe seal in the common iliac artery. The diameter of the iliac limb ranges from 8 to 24 mm, and the length ranges from 37 to 122 mm; the sizes available for the delivery introducer systems are 14F, 16F, and 18F. The outside diameter of the endograft is intended to be 10–15% larger than the proximal infrarenal aortic neck and the iliac arteries to provide an adequate seal and to reduce the risk of a type I endoleak. Proximal aortic and distal iliac extension

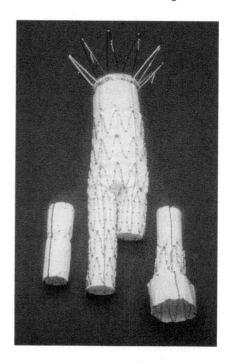

**Figure 12.1** The bifurcated Zenith AAA endovascular graft (Cook, Inc.) is a three-piece modular unit.

pieces are available, usually for the purpose of treating type I endoleaks or common iliac artery aneurysms [3]. The Zenith AAA endovascular graft is designed to provide longitudinal columnar support throughout the length of the graft to improve fixation and decrease kinking, twisting, and migration [3].

## Inclusion and exclusion requirements

Proximal and distal fixation is an important issue for any graft used in endovascular AAA repair. Current anatomical exclusion criteria for the Zenith device are the following: (1) significant occlusive disease, tortuosity, or calcification in the iliac vessels, making access difficult and dangerous, and (2) circumferential thrombus or atheroma within the proximal neck because of concerns about long-term integrity of the aortic wall and the potential for inadequate proximal fixation. Inclusion criteria are the following: (1) the proximal aortic neck must have a length that is ≥15 mm and a diameter that is 18–28 mm, (2) to avoid potential migration and problems with proximal fixation of the main body, the angle of the proximal aortic neck relative to the long axis of the aneurysm must be <60°, and the angle of the suprarenal neck relative to the infrarenal neck must be ≤45°, (3) the length of the iliac artery landing zone must be ≥10 mm, and (4) the diameter of the native common iliac artery must be 7.5–20 mm at the distal fixation site.

## Preoperative imaging

The anatomical assessment of the aorta and the iliac artery is key to deploying the stent graft safely and to decreasing the risk of type I and type III endoleaks. Thus, adequate preoperative imaging is crucial. Preoperative, high-resolution spiral computed tomographic images with 3-mm cuts are needed from the level of the superior mesenteric artery to the iliac bifurcation to measure accurately the aortic and iliac diameters and to identify thrombi, calcifications, and the shape of the proximal and distal landing zones. Three-dimensional reconstruction images may provide additional length and proximal angle measurements. Any uncertainty, however, especially in determining iliac dimensions, should be addressed with conventional angiography.

## Procedure

Before the procedure, as the size and length of the actual graft and its components are selected, one iliac system is designated as the "ipsilateral" side and the other as the "contralateral" side. The ipsilateral side is usually the larger and straighter side of the iliac system through which the large main body is delivered.

Bilateral femoral artery cutdowns are used. The contralateral femoral artery is punctured, and a guidewire (i.e., Bentson guidewire, Cook, Inc.) is advanced under fluoroscopic guidance into the suprarenal aorta. A 9F sheath is placed and a 5F pigtail angiographic catheter is passed over the guidewire to just above the renal arteries. After removal of the guidewire, the ipsilateral femoral artery is cannulated and a Bentson guidewire is passed up into the suprarenal aorta under fluoroscopic guidance. A 5F vertebral catheter is passed over the guidewire, and the guidewire is exchanged for a stiffer guidewire (i.e., Lunderquist guidewire, Cook, Inc.). Next the vertebral catheter is removed. Prior to insertion of the main body, the endograft should be properly oriented. The graft system should be rotated under fluoroscopy so that the contralateral limb radiopaque marker is positioned anterolaterally. In the correct anterolateral position the marker resembles a check mark (Figure 12.2). The main body is then passed over the Lunderquist guidewire under fluoroscopic guidance into the suprarenal aorta. Prior to graft deployment, using the pigtail angiographic catheter from the contralateral side, an arteriogram is obtained to identify the origins of the renal arteries.

After the level of the most distal renal artery has been accurately marked, the main body is unsheathed to position the covered portion of the endograft just distal to the renal arteries. The sheath is withdrawn until the contralateral gate is released, at which time the angiographic catheter is exchanged for a glide wire and a vertebral catheter. Both the glide wire and the vertebral catheter are withdrawn until they are just distal to the contralateral gate. The guidewire is then advanced into the gate, up into the main body of the device.

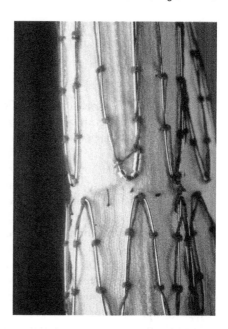

**Figure 12.2** Correctly positioned, the radiopaque marker in the contralateral limb resembles a check mark.

Next the vertebral catheter is passed over the guidewire up into the main body, and hand-injection angiography is performed to confirm that the contralateral gate has actually been cannulated. The proximal trigger wire is then removed and the proximal nose cone advanced to uncover the proximal bare stent crossing the renal arteries into the suprarenal aorta.

The contralateral vertebral catheter and glide wire are advanced through the bare stent into the suprarenal aorta. The guidewire is then exchanged for an Amplatz Super-Stiff guidewire (Cook, Inc.). Retrograde hand-injection angiography is performed after fluoroscopic positioning of the gate and the pelvis in the same field. The origin of the hypogastric artery is then confirmed and marked. The sheath is removed and the 14F to 18F contralateral delivery introducer system is passed into the external iliac artery. The contralateral stent graft is passed up through the gate of the main body so that there is at least one stent length of overlap within the gate and that distally the contralateral limb terminates at least 1 cm within the common iliac artery. The contralateral stent graft is then deployed.

After deployment of the contralateral graft, the remainder of the ipsilateral iliac end of the main body is unsheathed until the most distal stent has expanded. Next the distal stent trigger wire is released, and the nose cone is captured and withdrawn. A "molding balloon" (30-mm latex balloon, Cook, Inc.) is used to gently dilate the proximal aortic stent, all areas of stent graft overlap, and the distal attachment sites. Finally, completion aortography is performed to document patency of the graft and to rule out the presence of endoleaks. Type I endoleaks are treated at the time of implantation with repeated angioplasty and proximal or distal extensions as needed.

## Results

Stanley *et al.* (1) have reported on 238 patients treated with a Zenith bifurcated endovascular graft between 1994 and 1998. The only selection criterion that was found to be associated with migration was an aortic neck diameter larger than 28 mm. Type I endoleaks were four times more frequent in patients who had a proximal aortic neck length of <20 mm. There was no increased risk of distal type I endoleaks associated with iliac diameter. Proximal aortic neck contour changes, such as plaques of >3 mm, an inverted tunnel configuration, or a proximal aortic neck diameter of >28 mm, were also found to be predictive of the development of type I endoleaks.

Resch *et al.* [4] reported on 158 patients treated with Ivancev–Malmö monoiliac stent grafts (75 patients), Chuter bifurcated stent grafts (15 patients), Vanguard stent grafts (Boston Scientific Corp., Natick, MA) (15 patients), and Zenith stent grafts (53 patients). Patients in the Zenith and Vanguard groups had a lower risk of secondary interventions than patients in the other two groups. In the Vanguard and Zenith groups, the conversion, mortality, and distal migration rates were zero. Although follow-up has been relatively small for the bifurcated Zenith graft, >80% of the postoperative complications occurred within 18 months [4].

Greenberg *et al.* [2] reported on the early and mid-term results in 528 patients treated with the original Zenith device, which did not have the proximal transrenal bare stent with barbs. The patients were treated in seven institutions worldwide: 295 patients in Australia, 127 in European centers, and 106 in the United States. For 57% of the patients, mean follow-up was 14 months (range, 0–36 months). Complications associated with the initial implantation procedure were endoleaks in 15% of the patients; inability to obtain femoral access, requiring iliac access, in 14%; and cardiovascular complications in 7%. Extension pieces were required in 5.5%. Type I endoleaks were universally treated and type II endoleaks were selectively treated. During the follow-up period, 48 patients (9%) died. Two of these deaths (2 of 48; 4%) were related to aneurysmal rupture. Migration, defined as >5 mm of longitudinal movement with respect to the renal arteries, occurred in 14% of the patients during a 2- to 3-year follow-up [2].

The high rate of device migration necessitated a change in the Zenith endograft design. Experimental studies have demonstrated that a sutured graft anastomosis provides stronger fixation of the graft to the artery wall than any presently available stent. Self-expandable stents with hooks or barbs have provided better fixation than self-expandable stents without hooks or barbs [5]. Lambert *et al.* [6] showed in an experimental study on animal cadavers that stent fixation depends on the length of contact between the stent and the aortic wall. From this experimental work, the Zenith endograft design was changed to incorporate a proximal bare stent with barbs to allow transrenal fixation. Balloon dilatation of the proximal bare stent helps to anchor the barbs through the aortic wall after deployment. In the experience of Greenberg [3] with 250 Zenith devices that had a proximal aortic bare stent, there was no evidence of distal migration.

Several investigators have shown that there is no increased risk of renal impairment after transrenal stent placement [7–9]. Burks et al. [10] have reported on their experience with aortic endografts using two devices (Talent, Medtronic Inc., Minneapolis, MN, and Parodi/Palmaz). Transrenal fixation occurred in 49% of the patients. The uncovered stent was at or proximal to the level of the superior mesenteric artery in 95 of 192 patients. After a mean follow-up time of 25 months, none of the patients had an adverse event related to transrenal or suprarenal fixation. The serum creatinine levels remained stable and there was no evidence of renal, hepatic, splenic, or intestinal infarction on the postimplantation contrast-enhanced spiral computed tomographic scans. None of the 192 patients had a type I endoleak, and no migration was observed. Parodi & Ferreira [11] reported that the bare stent segment is covered by a layer of myointimal hyperplasia and becomes a part of the arterial wall, avoiding the problem of migration.

In our experience with 51 Zenith grafts deployed between April 2000 and December 2004, there were no conversions to open repair. One patient had a suprarenal aneurysm adjacent to the bare stent at 3 months. One late stent graft migration that occurred without an associated type I endoleak was caused by significant aortic neck dilatation, from 25 to 34 mm, 3 months after implantation. Open surgery was performed, and the visceral aorta was replaced with a distal anastomosis to the proximal end of the stent graft. Three type II endoleaks without enlargement of the aneurysm sac are under observation. One patient was treated for bilateral type IIIa endoleaks with additional endovascular components.

## Conclusion

The Zenith device has successfully completed phase 1 of the US Food and Drug Administration (FDA) trials, attesting to its safety. In November 1999, the FDA approved proceeding with a phase 2 trial with the intention to treat patients with abdominal aortic, aortoiliac, or iliac aneurysms. A prospective multicenter clinical study, involving 15 institutions in the United States, was initiated as part of the phase 2 FDA trial in January 2000 to compare the safety and effectiveness of the Zenith AAA endovascular graft with the safety and effectiveness of open aneurysm repair. The advantages of this device over currently available FDA-approved aortic endograft devices include suprarenal fixation, customization of size and length of the aortic stent graft, the ability to treat aneurysms with proximal neck diameters of up to 28 mm, and a low-profile delivery system. This trial will yield data on the efficacy of this device.

# References

1 Stanley BM, Semmens JB, Mai Q *et al*. Evaluation of patient selection guidelines for endoluminal AAA repair with the Zenith Stent-Graft: the Australasian experience. *J Endovasc Ther* 2001; **8**: 457–64.
2 Greenberg RK, Lawrence-Brown M, Bhandari G *et al*. An update of the Zenith endovascular graft for abdominal aortic aneurysms: initial implantation and mid-term follow-up data. *J Vasc Surg* 2001; **33**(Suppl): S157–64.
3 Greenberg RK. Abdominal aortic endografting: fixation and sealing. *J Am Coll Surg* 2002; 194 Suppl: S79–87.
4 Resch T, Malina M, Lindblad B, Ivancev K. The impact of stent-graft development on outcome of AAA repair: a 7-year experience. *Eur J Vasc Endovasc Surg* 2001; **22**: 57–61.
5 Resch T, Malina M, Lindblad B, Malina J, Brunkwall J, Ivancev K. The impact of stent design on proximal stent-graft fixation in the abdominal aorta: an experimental study. *Eur J Vasc Endovasc Surg* 2000; **20**: 190–5.
6 Lambert AW, Williams DJ, Budd JS, Horrocks M. Experimental assessment of proximal stent-graft (InterVascular) fixation in human cadaveric infrarenal aortas. *Eur J Vasc Endovasc Surg* 1999; **17**: 60–5.
7 Marin ML, Parsons RE, Hollier LH *et al*. Impact of transrenal aortic endograft placement on endovascular graft repair of abdominal aortic aneurysms. *J Vasc Surg* 1998; **28**: 638–46.
8 Bove PG, Long GW, Zelenock GB *et al*. Transrenal fixation of aortic stent-grafts for the treatment of infrarenal aortic aneurysmal disease. *J Vasc Surg* 2000; **32**: 697–703.
9 Malina M, Brunkwall J, Ivancev K, Lindh M, Lindblad B, Risberg B. Renal arteries covered by aortic stents: clinical experience from endovascular grafting of aortic aneurysms. *Eur J Vasc Endovasc Surg* 1997; **14**: 109–13.
10 Burks JA Jr, Faries PL, Gravereaux EC, Hollier LH, Marin ML. Endovascular repair of abdominal aortic aneurysms: stent-graft fixation across the visceral arteries. *J Vasc Surg* 2002; **35**: 109–13.
11 Parodi JC, Ferreira LM. Ten-year experience with endovascular therapy in aortic aneurysms. *J Am Coll Surg* 2002; **194**(Suppl): S58–66.

# CHAPTER 13

# PowerLink stent graft system

**Edward B. Diethrich, MD**

## Introduction

Since 1991, when Dr Juan Parodi published his report of a successful endoluminal graft exclusion of an abdominal aortic aneurysm (AAA) [1], endoluminal graft technology has advanced considerably. Although early studies demonstrated that the prototype straight tube graft designs without distal stent fixation were unsatisfactory, the work of Dr Parodi and other investigators pioneered successful interventional devices that have been used to treat thousands of patients who had AAAs.

The first commercially available bifurcated endoluminal graft was the MinTec device (MinTec, Inc., Laciotat, France), which was sold in Europe. Boston Scientific Corporation (Natick, MA) purchased and redesigned the device and reintroduced it in Europe under the name Stentor and later as Vanguard. A growing number of manufacturers have stepped into the endoluminal graft market, and various devices have received European Commission approval and are being sold outside the United States.

The regulatory process moves considerably slower in the United States. Investigational device exemptions are necessary before clinical assessment of devices can begin, and US Food and Drug Administration (FDA) approval generally takes several years. The first two commercial products approved in the United States were the Ancure device by Guidant Corporation/EndoVascular Technologies, Incorporated (Menlo Park, CA) and the AneuRx device by Medtronic AVE (Santa Rosa, CA). Both companies took their products to the FDA panel on the same day, and both received approval in September 1999. Approval for the Ancure device was withdrawn in 2003 because of unresolved issues with the delivery system. The Excluder graft (W.L. Gore and Associates, Inc., Flagstaff, AZ) and the Zenith graft (Cook, Inc., Bloomington, IN) were approved in 2002. The PowerLink AAA stent graft (Endologix, Inc., Irvine, CA) received FDA approval in October 2004.

Although there are no results yet from long-term trials for any of the endoluminal grafts on the market, various clinical difficulties have been encountered. Reported problems include erosion of the graft fabric, fractures of stents and grafts, perforations, endoleaks, and ruptures of the treated aneurysm. Rupture is the most serious of these complications, and in the United States, the problem has been reported in a small number of patients treated with the AneuRx graft. In the majority of cases, rupture has been associated with the phase 1 devices, which had a stiff bifurcated design. Rupture associated with the Ancure unibody device has been rare, but this complication has certainly dampened enthusiasm for endoluminal graft technology.

The Vascular Surgery Department at the Arizona Heart Institute and Arizona Heart Hospital (Phoenix, AZ) has been involved in endoluminal grafting for more than a decade. The institution obtained a single-center investigational device exemption, and protocols were approved by the FDA and the institution's investigational review board. My colleagues and I try to optimize our patient selection criteria, in part by evaluating success rates with available devices and studying complications.

After our early results with Dacron grafts (DuPont, Wilmington, DE) supported on either end by Palmaz stents (Cordis Corp., Miami, FL) were disappointing, we turned our research efforts to polytef-covered devices that were either partially or fully supported by a stent. These devices were the basis for the design of the current PowerLink prosthesis, which is fully supported and incorporates a polytef-covered stainless steel stent. Although the grafts were initially custom-made at our campus, the complexity of the delivery system eventually required us to enlist the help of a team of engineers and designers to further improve the design and production of the Power-Link stent graft.

This chapter reviews patient selection for AAA procedures and complications of AAA procedures, and it describes the PowerLink stent graft and our early clinical results.

## Assessing the appropriateness of the endovascular procedure

The decision to perform an endovascular procedure rather than an open surgical procedure must be weighed carefully. At present, there are no clear standards to guide the decision. If patients are considered at high risk for open surgical intervention, the endovascular procedure may be a reasonable alternative. Unfortunately, the appeal of offering endovascular procedures to those with serious comorbidities may be overshadowed by the potential for unsatisfactory results. In one study that reported outcomes of endoluminal graft implantation, the cumulative 1-year survival rates for patients considered to be unfit for open surgery or general anesthesia were only 20% and 23%, respectively [2].

The success of the endovascular procedure depends on various factors. Thorough clinical assessment and imaging are key in determining which patients are best suited for the procedure. It seems that men and patients with less tortuous arteries are often the best candidates. In a study of the Ancure and Talent (Medtronic, Inc., Minneapolis, MN) grafts, 141 patients were evaluated (19 women and 122 men) [3]. After identifying unsuitable anatomical features, investigators rejected 63.2% of the women but only 33.6% of the men ($P$ = 0.026). In another study, aortoiliac tortuosity was associated with increased complexity of endovascular repair; tortuosity of the aorta neck, in particular, was seen as a possible cause of early endoleaks [4]. These factors were considered during the design of the PowerLink prosthesis.

There are some data to suggest that morbidity may be less in elective endoluminal graft repair of AAAs than in elective open surgical repair. In one study [5], 250 patients with infrarenal AAAs were treated with the AneuRx stent graft ($n$ = 190) or with open repair ($n$ = 60), and those who received endovascular treatment had significantly less blood loss, less time to extubation, and fewer days in the intensive care unit and hospital. Major morbidity was 23% in the surgical group and 12% in the stent graft group ($P$ < 0.05).

In another study, the use of a low-profile, fully supported, modular, second-generation endoprosthesis ($n$ = 148) was compared with open repair ($n$ = 135) during the same period. The difference in perioperative mortality rates between the endoluminal graft group (2.7%) and the open repair group (5.9%) was not statistically significant [6]. Survival curves did show that the endoluminal graft group was favored ($P$ = 0.004), and a Kaplan-Meier curve for graft failure showed that 3-year success probabilities were similar between the two groups (82% in the endoluminal graft group and 85% in the open repair group).

In a separate evaluation ($N$ = 104), the 30-day perioperative mortality rate was 7.8% for "increased-risk" patients and 1.9% for "low-risk" patients ($P$ = not significant) [7]. Overall, clinical success rates were comparable in both patient groups; however, 2 years after endovascular repair was performed, at least 25% of the cases were classified as a clinical failure. In another study, morbidity and mortality were higher in patients treated with endoluminal grafts than in those who underwent an open surgical procedure [8]. Although these results included learning curve data, it is difficult to justify endovascular intervention in patients who are ideal candidates for open surgical repair. In studies of the PowerLink device, all candidates were accepted if their lesions were anatomically suited for device deployment; however, there are certainly no data that offer scientific justification for this stance.

## Complications associated with endovascular procedures

The propensity for endoleak is the Achilles heel of current endoluminal graft technology. Indeed, endoleaks—which are caused by incomplete exclusion of the aneurysm—are the most common complication associated with endoluminal grafting. Anatomical variations, the type of graft used, and the method of insertion all influence the endoleak rate [9]. Endoleaks include the following types: type I—related to graft attachment; type II—retrograde flow from collateral branches (called a retroleak); type III—fabric tears, graft disconnection, or graft disintegration; type IV—flow through the graft wall because of porosity [10]. Recent improvements in endoluminal prostheses have virtually eliminated type IV endoleaks.

A meta-analysis of 23 studies and 1189 patients described endoleaks associated with endovascular treatment of AAAs [11]. Among the 1118 patients who received transfemoral endoluminal grafts, endoleaks developed in 270. The most frequent site of endoleak was the distal stent attachment (36%); the most frequent time of occurrence was immediately after the procedure (66%); and the most frequent fate of the endoleaks was persistence over time (37%). Tube grafts were affected more frequently by endoleaks than bifurcated grafts ($P = 0.004$), and self-expandable grafts were associated with more endoleaks than balloon-expandable grafts ($P = 0.037$).

In a large ($N = 899$) multicenter trial [12], bifurcated devices were used in 91% of the patients, straight tube grafts in 7%, and aorto-uni-iliac devices in 2%. Clinical follow-up and computed tomographic studies were performed, and life table analyses were used to calculate the rates of freedom from persistent endoleak. Median follow-up was 6.2 months. Freedom from persistent endoleak was 93% at 6 months and 90% at 18 months. The 18-month cumulative patient survival was 88%. In patients with temporary endoleaks, the maximal transverse diameter was smaller at 6–12 months than at baseline. In patients with persistent endoleaks, the maximal transverse diameter at 6–12 months was no different than at baseline.

The association of endoleak and rupture remains unclear at this time. Whereas some investigators have demonstrated a lack of correlation [13], others believe there is indeed a relationship between these two factors [14]. Additional research suggests that endotension is an "indiscernible" low-flow endoleak [15] and that "freedom from endoleak" incorrectly suggests freedom from endotension [16], which may be a risk factor for rupture.

The potential for development of endoleaks may be predicted in some cases. In a group of patients treated with AneuRx grafts, Cox proportional hazards regression analysis showed that patent internal mesenteric arteries ($P < 0.01$) and patent lumbar arteries ($P < 0.0001$) were independent risk factors for persistent endoleaks and that persistent type II endoleaks were associated with an increase in AAA size and no significant change in the infrarenal neck diameter [17]. The contour, length, and diameter of the aneurysm neck are thought to be related to the risk of endoleaks [18]. If the contour of the neck changes by >3 mm ($P = 0.003$) or if the neck or aneurysm is <20 mm long ($P = 0.04$) or <10 mm wide ($P = 0.003$), the risk of endoleak at the proximal attachment site is significantly increased; each of these variables is affected by increased angulation. Aneurysms with dimensions that meet these criteria are not likely to be amenable to successful endovascular repair.

My colleagues and I have studied the relationship between endoleak and aneurysm sac pressures in the perioperative period after endovascular repair, and we have developed an algorithm to help detect endoleaks (Sharma R, Diethrich EB, Ramaiah V, Rodriguez J, Rosenthal D, read at the International

Congress XIV on Endovascular Interventions, Scottsdale, AZ, February 11–15, 2001). Continued pressure within the aneurysm sac after AAA endografting may cause expansion and aneurysmal rupture, but a decrease in the mean aneurysm sac pulse pressure to <20 mmHg and an endoleak ratio (arterial pulse pressure divided by the sac pulse pressure) >2.0 allow confirmation of the absence of an endoleak. Additional study is required to further document the success of this test in detecting endoleaks associated with AAA endoluminal grafting.

The treatment of endoleaks may require conversion to open surgical repair or insertion of a new stent or graft; however, both primary and secondary conversion have a high operative mortality rate [19]. When endoleaks are short and wide (types I and III), it is usually necessary to deploy another prosthesis or perform a surgical conversion [20]. When the endoleak has a patent channel that is long and narrow (type II), inducing thrombosis is often a successful means of treating the problem. Type II endoleaks may also be treated with a liquid embolic agent containing an ethylene-vinyl-alcohol copolymer [21]. The liquid is injected into the endoleak sac, and early results indicate that, in most cases, the copolymer provides a complete, durable occlusion.

## The PowerLink graft

### Design rationale

The advantages and disadvantages of current endoluminal graft configurations are being debated worldwide—a discussion that is likely to continue for several years. A few points about the design rationale for the PowerLink graft are worthy of comment. The delivery system for the prosthesis was intended to be user-friendly. Complexity in delivery systems seems only to enhance the opportunity for failure. A unibody graft configuration is appealing because it is simple and it minimizes modular attachment site problems. It also allows the device to rest on the bifurcation, rather than having the body of the graft float within the aneurysm sac. So far, the success of these design features has not been adequately confirmed and questions about the need for suprarenal fixation remain. At present, one configuration of the PowerLink graft incorporates suprarenal fixation (Figure 13.1), and early results are encouraging. As yet, the graft does not have hooks, barbs, or other anchoring features; future configurations may incorporate them.

The PowerLink graft is self-expanding and lends itself well to both cephalad and caudad postdeployment ballooning, should the need arise. Recrossing a limb or the body of the graft with a "J" wire or other flexible wire is not a problem. Suprarenal cuffs and limb extenders provide additional assurance of successful exclusion of the aneurysm. Straight aortic tube grafts and an aorto-uni-iliac configuration with a contralateral iliac excluder complete the array of devices presently available (Figure 13.2).

Delivery of the unibody bifurcated system has generally been accomplished by open exposure of one common femoral artery and percutaneous deploy-

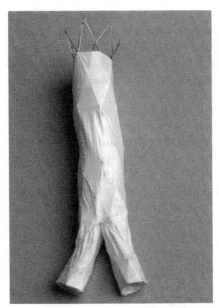

**Figure 13.1** At present, one configuration of the PowerLink graft (Endologix, Inc.) incorporates suprarenal fixation; the US Food and Drug Administration has approved study of this device in phase 2 trials.

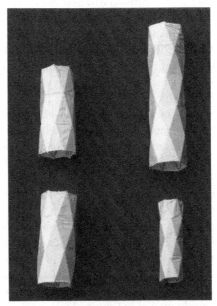

**Figure 13.2** Straight aortic tube grafts (upper left and lower left) and an aorto-uni-iliac configuration (upper right) with a contralateral iliac excluder (lower right) are available with the PowerLink graft (Endologix, Inc.).

ment of the contralateral limb. A few bifurcated systems have also been deployed percutaneously, as have the aortic tube grafts. The aorto-uni-iliac design requires bilateral exposure to the common femoral artery to complete the procedure with a femorofemoral bypass graft.

### Insertion of the PowerLink graft

The common femoral artery is exposed through an oblique incision just caudad to the inguinal ligament. If the common femoral artery is small, the external iliac artery is exposed caudad to the inguinal ligament and used for entry of the delivery device. A 12.5F peel-away sheath (SafeSheath, Pressure Products, Inc., Rancho Palos Verdes, CA) is inserted. The opposite common femoral artery is cannulated with a 9F sheath. Heparin (5000 units) is injected intravenously. Contrast medium is injected bilaterally to assess the iliac arteries, the origin and nature of the internal iliac arteries, and the degree of iliac tortuosity. Bilateral 0.035-inch angled Glidewires (Medi-tech/Boston Scientific Corp., Natick, MA) are passed into the lower abdominal aorta, and a Microvena snare (Microvena Corp., White Bear Lake, MN) is used to pull either Glidewire (it does not matter which one) to the appropriate sheath, where it exits (Figure 13.3a).

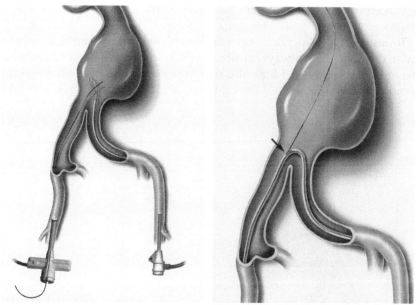

a                                                                                          b

**Figure 13.3** (a) A snare is used to pull one of the guidewires to the appropriate sheath, where it exits. As shown here, the irrigation port on the delivery sheath of the PowerLink device (Endologix, Inc.) should always point toward the contralateral side. (b) A crossover catheter is passed from the contralateral to the ipsilateral side to eliminate any possibility of the contralateral pull wire and the main delivery wire becoming entangled. The catheter is positioned so that the hole (arrow), marked by radiopaque beads, is located at about the 11-o'clock position on the fluoroscopic screen.

An aortogram is performed using a pigtail catheter. The image intensifier is positioned so that the renal arteries are seen at the top of the fluoroscopic screen and the crossover wire is seen below them. An optional step is to place a needle transversely on the skin to identify the level of the renal arteries. After the image is obtained, the image intensifier is not moved, thereby eliminating the problem of parallax. A crossover catheter is passed from the left (contralateral) to the right (ipsilateral) side (Figure 13.3b). The catheter is positioned so that the hole, marked by radiopaque beads, is located at about the 11-o'clock position on the fluoroscopic screen. This ensures that the stiff wire (nitinol guidewire; Microvena Corp.), over which the prosthesis is delivered, can pass into the suprarenal position through the hole in the crossover catheter.

The PowerLink device is placed on the table and prepared for delivery. The stiff delivery wire is passed through the device, and the contralateral pull wire is loaded into the crossover catheter and pulled through until it appears on the opposite side. The crossover catheter is removed while the crossover wire is held firmly at its junction on the delivery sheath; this prevents premature disconnection of the wire and contralateral limb. The prosthesis is advanced to the common femoral artery sheath. The sheath is withdrawn, and the common femoral artery is squeezed between the thumb and index finger to prevent bleeding while the peel-away sheath is removed. The prosthesis is advanced into the common femoral artery as the contralateral pull wire is pulled gently.

To ensure proper alignment from the contralateral sheath and to avoid wire twist, the pull wire is always oriented medially and the guidewire laterally at the level of the groin. Additionally, the irrigation port on the delivery sheath should always point toward the contralateral side (Figure 13.4). Under fluo-

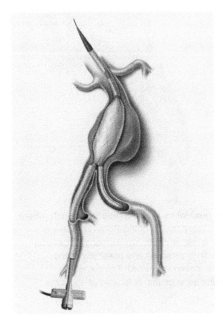

**Figure 13.4** Deployment of the PowerLink graft (Endologix, Inc.). The nose cone is positioned above the renal arteries; the main body has been released up to the most proximal stent, which is positioned just below the renal arteries. The contralateral limb is in place for release and the ipsilateral limb is still contained within the sheath.

roscopic control, the prosthesis is delivered above the aortic bifurcation. The contralateral pull wire is withdrawn into the left groin to remove excess slack. The contralateral limb is freed by retracting its retaining sheath while the contralateral pull wire is gently pulled from the groin. The main body of the prosthesis is resheathed. The cephalad end of the graft is lowered and positioned at the level of the renal artery. The body of the graft is deployed up to the most cephalad stent. The deployment is caudad to cephalad.

Until the body is completely deployed by releasing the most cephalad stent, the graft can be moved in relation to the renal arteries. The prosthesis is held in position as the contralateral pull wire is pulled to release the contralateral limb, and the last stent is released to complete the deployment of the main body. The push rod is advanced farther until it encapsulates the nose cone. The nose cone is withdrawn through the body of the graft to the ipsilateral limb, which is still covered by the sheath. The ipsilateral limb is deployed, and the nose cone is withdrawn into the sheath; the entire assembly is removed. A 9F sheath is inserted into the right common femoral artery, and a control angiogram is obtained. Bilateral femoral sheath angiography is performed to confirm the absence of a distal endoleak. The right common femoral artery is repaired. The incision is closed, and the patient is returned to the recovery unit; the left common femoral artery sheath is removed when the activated clotting time returns to the normal range.

## Early clinical results

Clinical trials of the PowerLink graft are currently in progress, and the most recent results were presented at the International Congress XVII on Endovascular Interventions (Scottsdale, AZ; February 2004). A total of 92 patients were treated in a single-center study from 1999 to 2003. The PowerLink graft was successfully deployed in 97% of the procedures, and there were no device-related deaths. The mean duration of the procedure was 91 min, and the average decrease in the diameter of the aneurysm sac was 44% at 3 months and 67% at 12 months. There were three early endoleaks (3.3%) and four late endoleaks (4.3%). At 36 months, 91% of the patients were free of endoleaks, and the cumulative survival rate was 95%. Results of an earlier multicenter study indicated similarities to the single-center study, with high technical success and low endoleak and morbidity and mortality rates [22].

## Case study

Although the investigative trials of the device are still under way, the results to date have been satisfactory. The graft and the deployment system are easy to use and are likely to have various indications in the future. The Arizona Heart Institute and Arizona Heart Hospital have a separate investigational device exemption that extends the indications for treatment with the device and allows the use of the PowerLink graft to treat patients who have a ruptured AAA. In one instance, for example, a patient arrived at the Arizona Heart Hospital by air ambulance approximately 6 h after her AAA ruptured and caused a massive retroperitoneal hemorrhage (Figure 13.5a,b). The

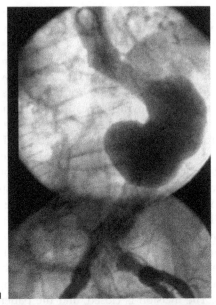

a

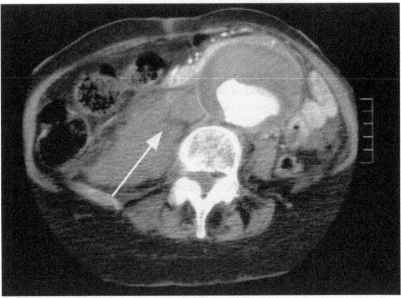

b

**Figure 13.5** (a) Intraoperative aortogram in a patient with acute rupture of an abdominal aortic aneurysm (AAA). (b) Computed tomographic scan shows massive retroperitoneal hemorrhage and rupture of the AAA (arrow).

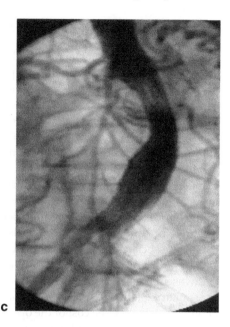

**Figure 13.5** *Continued* (c) Control angiogram shows immediate sealing of the ruptured AAA. Only 36 min elapsed from the initiation of local anesthesia to the completed percutaneous delivery of the prosthesis.

**c**

angiogram showed an 8-cm infrarenal aneurysm. It was possible to treat this patient percutaneously using the PowerLink graft, and a bifurcated device was deployed within 40 min of her arrival in the endovascular suite (Figure 13.5c). Although rupture of an AAA is frequently fatal, rapid treatment yielded an excellent result in this patient.

## The future of endoluminal grafting

As the search continues for optimal solutions to treat vascular disease, it seems that new technology will become increasingly important. Minimally invasive endoluminal procedures, in particular, hold great appeal. Short-term technical success with endovascular AAA treatment is high, and significant reductions in operating time, length of intensive care unit stay, and length of hospital stay have been realized in comparisons with open surgical resection. In addition, improvements in device design and deployment techniques have brought routine success with these procedures closer. Still, a perfect device has yet to be developed.

In an effort to improve clinical results with endovascular procedures, several investigators are studying new stents and grafts that incorporate vehicles to administer pharmacologic agents or provide cell seeding or gene therapy technology. Antiproliferative agents, such as paclitaxel and rapamycin, are being delivered in polymer carriers to decrease the incidence of neointimal hyperplasia. Endoluminal grafts incorporating stents with new, thromboresistant metals are also under study, as are those that possess biomembrane coatings such as phosphorylcholine or antithrombotic agents such as heparin.

Although advances in endovascular device technology may eventually limit complications associated with percutaneous procedures, the ultimate decision by the individual practitioner or the institutional team about the choice between endovascular technology and open surgical intervention is not a simple one. Skill level, operator experience, ability to treat life-threatening emergencies, commitment to long-term surveillance, and afford-ability of the procedure are only some of the considerations that must be weighed in assessing each case.

Indeed, cost is an important consideration. At present, the price of an endo-luminal graft nearly exceeds the total US Medicare reimbursement allotted for the procedure. Until competition between device manufacturers decreases the price of equipment—which seems very unlikely in the near future—the expense associated with endoluminal grafts will continue to be a concern.

Despite the expense of endoluminal grafts, some initial comparisons of endovascular and open procedures indicate that the costs of these procedures are similar [23]. In one study, the overall cost of the endovascular therapy was about 14% less than the cost of the open procedure; the higher cost of the open procedure was related to longer intensive care unit and hospital stays [24]. Performing presurgical evaluations on an outpatient basis may further decrease the costs of endovascular procedures.

Like cost data, information about patients' quality of life and its relation to the benefits of endovascular surgery is limited. In one study [25], however, the benefit of endovascular AAA repair in quality-adjusted life-years was con-sistently greater than that of open repair. Among older patients in poor health, endovascular surgery decreased the optimal threshold diameter for elective AAA repair. In another study, patients treated with endovascular procedures had better physical and functional scores as early as 1 week after hospital dis-missal and also returned to baseline status significantly earlier than patients who had open procedures [26].

## Summary

Although >10 years have passed since the first published account of endolu-minal graft treatment of an AAA, endoluminal graft technology is still in a relatively early stage. Patient selection and the prevention and management of complications have improved considerably, and endoluminal graft designs have advanced appreciably. Nevertheless, the study of results with available devices and the consideration of ways to improve existing technology continue.

The self-expanding PowerLink graft incorporates several features that are important to the short-term and long-term success of endoluminal grafting. The delivery system for the prosthesis was designed to be user-friendly. A unibody graft configuration was chosen because it is simple and minimizes modular attachment-site problems. Suprarenal fixation is under study, and the feature has been incorporated into one configuration of the PowerLink graft.

Overall, results with the PowerLink graft have been quite good, with a very high rate of short-term technical success and a low rate of endoleaks. The graft has been used to repair emergent rupture, and the device's versatility and ease of use are impressive. Long-term follow-up is now particularly important in determining the ultimate success of the PowerLink graft and other devices that are currently available or are coming to market. Results of percutaneous intervention are encouraging, and careful study is expected to improve endoluminal graft technology in the future.

## References

1 Parodi JC, Palmaz JC, Barone HD. Transfemoral intraluminal graft implantation for abdominal aortic aneurysms. *Ann Vasc Surg* 1991; **5**: 491–9.

2 Laheij RJ, van Marrewijk CJ, for the EUROSTAR group. Endovascular stenting of abdominal aortic aneurysm in patients unfit for elective open surgery. *Lancet* 2000; **356**: 832.

3 Velazquez OC, Larson RA, Baum RA *et al.* Gender-related differences in infrarenal aortic aneurysm morphologic features: issues relevant to Ancure and Talent endografts. *J Vasc Surg* 2001; **33**(Suppl): S77–84.

4 Wolf YG, Tillich M, Lee WA *et al.* Impact of aortoiliac tortuosity on endovascular repair of abdominal aortic aneuryms: evaluation of 3D computer-based assessment. *J Vasc Surg* 2001; **34**: 594–9.

5 Treiman GS, Lawrence PF, Edwards WH Jr *et al.* An assessment of the current applicability of the EVT endovascular graft for treatment of patients with an infrarenal abdominal aortic aneurysm. *J Vasc Surg* 1999; **30**: 68–75.

6 May J, White GH, Waugh R *et al.* Improved survival after endoluminal repair with second-generation prostheses compared with open repair in the treatment of abdominal aortic aneurysms: a 5-year concurrent comparison using life table method. *J Vasc Surg* 2001; **33**(Suppl): S21–6.

7 Bush RL, Lumsden AB, Dodson TF *et al.* Mid-term results after endovascular repair of the abdominal aortic aneurysm. *J Vasc Surg* 2001; **33**(Suppl): S70–6.

8 Cohnert TU, Oelert F, Wahlers T *et al.* Matched-pair analysis of conventional versus endoluminal AAA treatment outcomes during the initial phase of an aortic endografting program. *J Endovasc Ther* 2000; **7**: 94–100.

9 White GH, May J, Waugh RC, Chaufour X, Yu W. Type III and type IV endoleak: toward a complete definition of blood flow in the sac after endoluminal AAA repair. *J Endovasc Surg* 1998; **5**: 305–9.

10 May J, White GH, Waugh R *et al.* Adverse events after endoluminal repair of abdominal aortic aneurysms: a comparison during two successive periods of time. *J Vasc Surg* 1999; **29**: 32–7.

11 Schurink GW, Aarts NJ, van Bockel JH. Endoleak after stent-graft treatment of abdominal aortic aneurysm: a meta-analysis of clinical studies. *Br J Surg* 1999; **86**: 581–7.

12 Cuypers P, Buth J, Harris PL, Gevers E, Lahey R. Realistic expectations for patients with stent-graft treatment of abdominal aortic aneurysms: results of a European multicentre registry. *Eur J Vasc Endovasc Surg* 1999; **17**: 507–16.

13 Zarins CK, White RA, Hodgson KJ, Schwarten D, Fogarty TJ. Endoleak as a predictor of outcome after endovascular aneurysm repair: AneuRx multicenter clinical trial. *J Vasc Surg* 2000; **32**: 90–107.

14 White RA, Donayre C, Walot I, Stewart M. Abdominal aortic aneurysm rupture following endoluminal graft deployment: report of a predictable event. *J Endovasc Ther* 2000; **7**: 257–62.

15 White GH, May J, Petrasek P *et al.* Endotension: an explanation for continued AAA growth after successful endoluminal repair. *J Endovasc Surg* 1999; **6**: 308–15.

16 Gilling-Smith GL, Martin J, Sudhindran S *et al.* Freedom from endoleak after endovascular aneurysm repair does not equal treatment success. *Eur J Vasc Endovasc Surg* 2000; **19**: 421–5.

17 Arko FR, Rubin GD, Johnson BL *et al.* Type-II endoleaks following endovascular AAA repair: preoperative predictors and long-term effects. *J Endovasc Ther* 2001; **8**: 503–10.

18 Stanley BM, Semmens JB, Mai Q *et al.* Evaluation of patient selection guidelines for endoluminal AAA repair with the Zenith stent-graft: the Australasian experience. *J Endovasc Ther* 2001; **8**: 457–64.

19 Cuypers PW, Laheij RJ, Buth J, the EUROSTAR Collaborators. Which factors increase the risk of conversion to open surgery following endovascular abdominal aortic aneurysm repair? *Eur J Vasc Endovasc Surg* 2000; **20**: 183–9.

20 Mehta M, Ohki T, Veith FJ, Lipsitz EC. All sealed endoleaks are not the same: a treatment strategy based on an *ex-vivo* analysis. *Eur J Vasc Endovasc Surg* 2001; **21**: 541–4.

21 Martin ML, Dolmatch BL, Fry PD, Machan LS. Treatment of type II endoleaks with Onyx. *J Vasc Interv Radiol* 2001; **12**: 629–32.

22 Hansen CJ, Aziz I, Kim BB, Donayre CE, White RA, Endologix Investigators. Results from the Endologix PowerLink multicenter trial. *Semin Vasc Surg* 2003; **16**: 166–70.

23 Berman SS, Gentile AT, Berens ES, Haskell J. Institutional economic losses associated with AAA repair are independent of technique. *J Endovasc Ther* 2002; **9**: 282–8.

24 Holzenbein J, Kretschmer G, Glanzl R *et al.* Endovascular AAA treatment: expensive prestige or economic alternative? *Eur J Vasc Endovasc Surg* 1997; **14**: 265–72.

25 Finlayson SR, Birkmeyer JD, Fillinger MF, Cronenwett JL. Should endovascular surgery lower the threshold for repair of abdominal aortic aneurysms? *J Vasc Surg* 1999; **29**: 973–85.

26 Aquino RV, Jones MA, Zullo TG, Missig-Carroll N, Makaroun MS. Quality of life assessment in patients undergoing endovascular or conventional AAA repair. *J Endovasc Ther* 2001; **8**: 521–8.

# PART III

## Investigational stent graft devices

# CHAPTER 14

# Lifepath AAA bifurcated graft system

**Sashi Kilaru, MD, K. Craig Kent, MD**

## Introduction

The Lifepath AAA bifurcated graft system (Edwards Lifesciences Corp., Irvine, CA) is a balloon-expandable, modular, aortic stent graft developed for the treatment of infrarenal abdominal aortic aneurysms (AAAs). This device is a direct adaptation of a prototype developed in 1993 by White and colleagues [1].

## Graft design

The Lifepath AAA bifurcated graft system is composed of three primary units: a bifurcated graft trunk and two iliac limbs (Figure 14.1). All components are balloon expandable, although the graft trunk contains a segment that is self-expanding. Each component is introduced through its own delivery system. The grafts are constructed from woven polyester fabric that is similar in composition and strength to the Dacron graft materials (DuPont, Wilmington, DE) currently used for open aneurysm repair. The wireforms are composed of annealed Elgiloy (Elgiloy Specialty Metals, Elgin, IL), which is a corrosion-resistant, fatigue-resistant alloy created from cobalt, chromium, nickel, and molybdenum.

The graft trunk has a straight proximal section (5 cm long) and two limbs (the ipsilateral limb extends 3.7 cm and the contralateral limb extends 2.5 cm below the bifurcation) (Figure 14.2). Thus, one of the requirements for use of the graft is that the distance from the renal arteries to the aortic bifurcation be at least 9.0 cm. The proximal portion of the trunk contains four independent wireforms: three are interwoven into the polyester graft matrix, and the fourth is sewn to the exterior of the graft with polyester suture. These top four wireforms provide for attachment of the main body of the graft to the proximal aorta. A fifth wireform, composed of heat-treated, spring-tempered, self-expanding Elgiloy, extends from the main body of the graft into the iliac limbs. This wireform supports the bifurcation of the graft, prevents kinking, and allows fluoroscopic visualization of the graft septum. Both limbs of the main graft contain balloon-expandable wireforms that are also made of Elgiloy. These wireforms provide support for the limbs, increase the force of attachment between the limbs and the iliac grafts, and aid in fluoroscopic

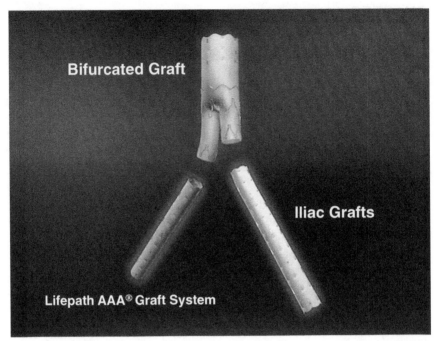

**Figure 14.1** Lifepath AAA graft system (Edwards Lifesciences Corp.) with main bifurcated graft trunk and iliac limbs.

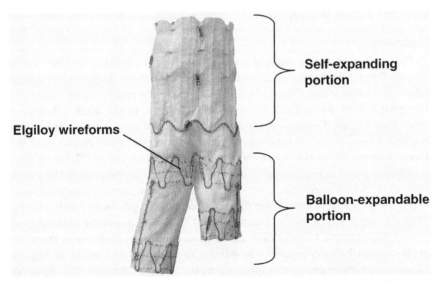

**Figure 14.2** Bifurcated graft trunk fully deployed (Elgiloy wireforms; Elgiloy Specialty Metal).

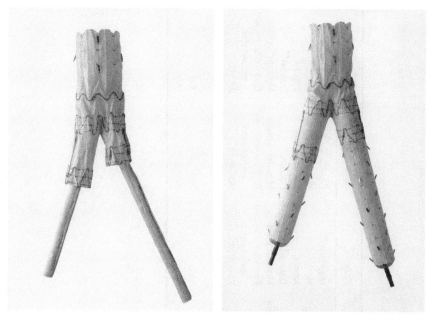

**Figure 14.3** Bifurcated main trunk with iliac limbs inserted (left) and fully balloon expanded (right).

visualization of the limbs. The wireforms of each limb are connected on the lateral side with a single longitudinal support wire made of Elgiloy. The wire contains a radiopaque marker. These longitudinal support wires are sewn to the exterior of the graft with a polyester suture.

The iliac grafts contain wireforms also made of Elgiloy. These wireforms are interwoven into the polyester graft matrix and placed throughout the length of each graft. The proximal portion of the iliac graft is anchored either within one of the limbs of the graft trunk or within another iliac limb (Figure 14.3). An overlap of at least 2 cm is recommended. The distal portion of the iliac limb is anchored into a nonaneurysmal iliac artery. The diameters of the balloons used for graft expansion range from 23 to 29 mm (main body) and from 12 to 16 mm (iliac limbs). The salient similarities and differences between the Lifepath AAA graft and other grafts are outlined in Table 14.1.

### Delivery system

The delivery system includes an introducer sheath and a graft delivery unit. In addition, a third unit, a directional catheter, facilitates wire placement through the contralateral limb of the main body of the graft (Figure 14.4). The dilator of the introducer sheath has a smooth tapered tip. One radiopaque marker is located near the tip, and a second radiopaque marker is located at

Table 14.1 Features of endovascular grafts.

| Feature | AneuRx | Quantum LP | PowerLink | Excluder | Talent | Zenith | Lifepath AAA |
|---|---|---|---|---|---|---|---|
| Manufacturer | Medtronic* | Cordis† | Endologix‡ | W.L. Gore§ | Medtronic* | Cook\|\| | Edwards¶ |
| FDA approval | Yes | No | Yes | Yes | No | Yes | No |
| Skeleton | Nitinol | Nitinol | Stainless steel | Nitinol | Nitinol | Stainless steel | Elgiloy# |
| Fabric | Dacron** | Dacron** | Polytef | Polytef | Dacron** | Dacron** | Dacron** |
| Body | Modular 2-piece | Modular 3-piece | Unibody | Modular 2-piece | Modular 2-piece | Modular 3-piece | Modular 3-piece |
| Construction | Exoskeleton | Endoskeleton | Endoskeleton | Exoskeleton | Endoskeleton and exoskeleton | Endoskeleton and exoskeleton | Endoskeleton and exoskeleton |
| Delivery size (ipsilateral/contralateral), F | 21/16 | 21/18 | 21/12 | 18/12 | 20–24/18 | 20/14–16 | 21/16 |
| Full support | Yes | Yes | Yes | Yes | Yes | Yes | Yes |
| Hooks/barbs | No | Yes | No | Yes | No | Yes | No |

FDA, US Food and Drug Administration.
*Medtronic, Inc., Minneapolis, MN.
†Cordis Corp., Miami, FL.
‡Endologix, Inc., Irvine, CA.
§W.L. Gore and Associates, Inc., Flagstaff, AZ.
\|\|Cook, Inc., Bloomington, IN.
¶Edwards Lifesciences Corp., Irvine, CA.
#Elgiloy Specialty Metals, Elgin, IL.
**DuPont, Wilmington, DE.

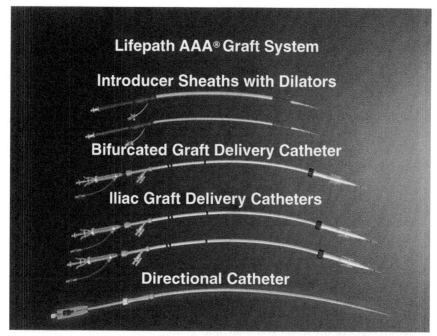

**Figure 14.4** Lifepath AAA graft system sheaths and delivery catheters (Edwards Lifesciences Corp.).

the tip of the sheath. The graft delivery unit consists of a graft loader, a polyester balloon, and a pusher. The endovascular graft and balloon are placed in the graft loader. The balloon is noncompliant and contains two radiopaque markers. The pusher abuts the compressed endovascular graft, eliminating movement during graft placement and allowing the release of the graft from the loader.

The directional catheter is a unique device that facilitates wire access to the contralateral limb (Figure 14.5). The catheter has two lumens. One allows the directional catheter to track over a 0.035-inch guidewire. The sheath of the directional catheter is then retracted, and its spring tip can be deflected by use of a knob located on its handle. A second 0.035-inch guidewire is passed through the other lumen of the catheter and exits through the deflecting tip, down the contralateral limb. The directional catheter is then removed, leaving wire access to the contralateral limb.

## Device deployment

Deployment of the Lifepath AAA bifurcated endovascular graft system consists of four steps:

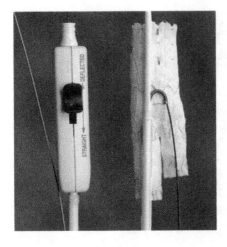

**Figure 14.5** Directional catheter in the deflected position allowing wire access into the contralateral limb.

1 deployment of the bifurcated main graft
2 contralateral guidewire access
3 deployment of the contralateral iliac limb graft
4 deployment of the ipsilateral iliac limb graft

## Deployment of the bifurcated main graft

Bilateral groin incisions are made to expose the femoral arteries, and 8F sheaths are inserted. After an aortogram is performed as necessary, a stiff guidewire is inserted into the descending thoracic aorta from the ipsilateral limb and the patient is systemically heparinized. The main introducer sheath is then placed over the guidewire so that its tip rests proximal to the level of the renal arteries. The dilator is removed, leaving the sheath in place. The graft delivery unit is then advanced into the sheath over the guidewire into the desired position. The introducer sheath is retracted, and angiography is used to confirm the location of the graft in relation to the renal arteries. At this step, the pusher may be rotated to allow for correct orientation of the graft. After the desired orientation and position are achieved, the graft is deployed by inflating the balloon to a maximum of 2 atm (202 kPa) for 30 s, and the balloon is removed.

## Contralateral guidewire access

The next step is to establish guidewire access into the contralateral limb. This is accomplished with the directional catheter as previously described. As the guidewire is advanced into the contralateral iliac artery, it is retrieved using a loop snare inserted from the contralateral groin. Care should be taken as the guidewire is removed from the contralateral sheath to avoid traction on the septum of the bifurcated graft. This guidewire is then exchanged for a stiff guidewire placed into the descending thoracic aorta.

## Deployment of the contralateral iliac limb graft

After the contralateral guidewire access has been established, a 16F introducer sheath is advanced over the guidewire into the contralateral limb of the main graft trunk. The graft loader containing the chosen contralateral iliac limb and associated balloon is then advanced over the guidewire into the sheath. This limb is then positioned to provide an overlap with the limb of the main graft of at least 2 cm. It is recommended that the iliac graft have a distal attachment zone of at least 1.5 cm within a segment of a nonaneurysmal iliac artery. The limb is then deployed by inflating the balloon to 5 atm (505 kPa) for 45 s.

## Deployment of the ipsilateral iliac limb graft

The directional catheter is removed, and the ipsilateral limb is advanced over the guidewire. This graft is similarly positioned with a 2-cm overlap within the ipsilateral limb of the main graft and with a 1.5-cm distal attachment. A kissing-balloon technique is used to simultaneously expand both iliac limbs. Completion angiography is then performed to assess patency of the graft and exclusion of the aneurysm.

## Device development

Prototypes of this device were initially evaluated by White and coworkers in canine models with various materials and graft configurations. An optimal version of the graft was created and clinical trials were begun by White & Yu in 1994. By 1996, a total of 112 implants had been performed using various devices, including straight, aorto-uni-iliac, and bifurcated grafts [1]. The final graft design was created with woven polyester graft material and wireforms composed of Elgiloy. A bifurcated graft was used in 27 of these patients, and all but the first four patients who were studied received devices that resemble the current Edwards Lifepath graft. This subset of 23 patients was followed up for as long as 3 years. The graft was successfully placed in 21 of 23 patients. In these 23 patients, the perioperative mortality was 4%. Retroperitoneal access to an iliac artery was required in four patients and repair of the femoral artery in two patients; wound infection occurred in one patient and graft thrombosis in one patient. The majority of these complications were thought to be associated with the relatively large diameter and lack of flexibility of the 24F internal and 29F external delivery sheaths. Other complications observed during the prototype clinical trial were myocardial infarction (two patients), unstable angina (one patient), stable angina (two patients), respiratory failure (two patients), and fever >38.5°C (eight patients). Endoleak was not found perioperatively in any of these 21 patients. Three late endoleaks were discovered (two type I, one type II) at 4, 6, and 24 months. Beyond the perioperative period, graft thrombosis or stenosis did not develop in any patient. No graft migration was reported. Aneurysm size decreased in all successfully treated cases [2].

After this trial, Baxter Healthcare Corporation (Deerfield, IL) and later Edwards Lifesciences Corporation began turning this "homemade" product into a commercially available device. Phase 1 and phase 2 trials were organized and implemented using straight as well as bifurcated grafts.

## Phase 1 and phase 2 studies

Inclusion and exclusion criteria for the trials are listed in Table 14.2. Computed tomography was required preoperatively as well as at the time of hospital discharge and at 6 months and 1, 2, and 3 years postoperatively.

The Straight Graft trial began in December 1996. Investigators at 24 sites entered 79 patients (male, 85%; mean age, 72 years). Of the 79 patients, 52 were test patients and 27 were control patients who underwent conventional surgical repair; 67 were available for evaluation at the time of this reporting [2]. In the test group, perioperative mortality was 0% and morbidity was 22%, including fever (>38.5°C: test patients, 16%; control patients, 23%), transfusion (test patients, 2%; control patients, 46%), and cardiac complications (test patients, 4%; control patients, 27%). The endoleak rate (any type of endoleak, as determined by the investigators) in the test patients was 14% (7 of 50) at 6 months and 20% (10 of 50) at 6 months to 3 years. One patient in the test group died of an expanding aneurysm that ruptured 33 months after implantation. This patient did not have a demonstrable endoleak on arteriography 2 months before the rupture.

The Bifurcated Graft trial began in December 1998 [3]. Of the 110 patients in this trial, 79 test patients (mean age, 68 years) received the bifurcated graft and 31 control patients (mean age, 70 years) underwent conventional open aneurysm repair; 94 were male and 16 were female. Follow-up was available in 100% of test patients. There were no perioperative deaths among test patients or control patients. In 4 of the 79 test patients the endograft could not be delivered or deployed. One aortic rupture occurred during graft deployment. Two of the 79 test patients (2.5%), inclusive of the patient who had the aortic rupture, required immediate conversion to open repair. Blood transfusions were required in 12 of the 79 test patients (15%) and in 29 of the 31 control patients (94%). A postoperative temperature >38.5°C occurred in 4% of the test patients and 6% of the control patients. The long-term mortality was 6% for the test group (5 of 79) and 3% for the control group (1 of 31). None of the deaths were related to the endovascular procedure or to aneurysmal rupture. There were no late ruptures. At 6 months, 4% of the test subjects (3 of 79) had an endoleak (two type I, one type II). Four of the 79 test patients (5%) had an endoleak at long-term follow-up (6 months to 3 years). Two patients required late conversion to open repair.

In April 2000, wireform fractures were found in two test patients, both of whom were asymptomatic. The data monitoring and safety subcommittee then convened and recommended suspension of further test patient enrollment in the trial. Consequently, effective April 2000, Edwards Lifesciences Corporation voluntarily suspended test patient enrollment for the Straight

**Table 14.2** Criteria for phase 1 and phase 2 studies.

**Inclusion criteria**
Medical inclusion criteria
• Age 40–85 years
• Availability for 3-year follow-up
• Saccular infrarenal AAA of any size or fusiform AAA >5 cm diameter or fusiform AAA with a diameter of 4–5 cm and at least one of the following:
  – Double the diameter of the normal aorta
  – Evidence of growth over 1 year >0.5 cm
  – Symptoms of back or abdominal pain associated with AAA
  – Age <65 years
  – Family history of aneurysm (first-degree or primary relative)
Anatomical inclusion criteria
• Proximal neck length ≥15 mm
• Proximal neck diameter 19–27 mm
• Renal-aortic bifurcation length ≥90 mm
• Proximal neck angulation <60°
• Nonaneurysmal attachment zone length >15 mm in common or external iliac artery
• Ipsilateral access arteries accommodate 25F OD delivery sheath; contralateral access artery accommodates 18F OD delivery sheath

**Exclusion criteria**
Medical exclusion criteria
• Female patient of childbearing potential
• Anesthesia risk group class IV or V
• Baseline creatinine level >2 mg/dL
• Treatment with another investigational device or drug
• Ruptured, leaking, or mycotic aneurysm
• Active infection
• Hemophilia or untreated bleeding diathesis
• Body weight >300 lb (136 kg)
• Marfan syndrome or other connective tissue disease
• Known allergy to all current radiologic contrast agents
Anatomical exclusion criteria
• Involvement of renal arteries
• Involvement of either internal iliac artery
• Accessory renal artery that would be covered by endograft
• Distal aortic lumen diameter <18 mm
• Iliac aneurysms beyond distal attachment zone
• Prior stent or endovascular graft
• Patent inferior mesenteric artery in association with a meandering mesenteric artery or a superior mesenteric artery occlusion
• Iliac artery tortuosity that, in the opinion of the investigator, will prevent passage of the access sheath

AAA, abdominal aortic aneurysm; OD, outer diameter.

Graft trial and the Bifurcated Graft trial. After further analysis, the wireform fracture rate for both the straight graft and the bifurcated graft studies was found to be 14.6% (13 of 89 patients) at 6 months, 21.9% (14 of 64) at 12 months, 34.8% (8 of 23) at 24 months, and 58.3% (7 of 12) at 3 years. Logistic regression analysis did not uncover a correlation between wireform fracture and clinical predictors, including patient age, sex, and weight; graft diameter, length, and angulation; aneurysm type; and preoperative hypertension. Endoleak rates in both studies were not significantly different between patients who had wireform fractures and those who did not. The long-term clinical consequence of these wireform fractures is unknown.

## Changes in graft design
In subsequent analyses the cause of wireform fractures seemed to be related to the curvature, the angle of peak, and the diameter of the wires. With this knowledge, the manufacturer created a second-generation graft with a new wireform structure designed to prevent fracture. The wire diameter in this second-generation graft is 25% larger, producing a nearly 50% decrease in compliance. Additional graft improvements in the second-generation device included increasing the diameter of the limbs of the aortic graft from 13 to 15 mm to facilitate balloon removal, and correspondingly increasing the diameter in the proximal end of the iliac graft from 14 to 16 mm. The new graft can be deployed through a smaller, 21F introducer that is fitted with a Kraton tip (Kraton Polymers, Houston, TX). With the new second-generation graft, Edwards Lifesciences Corporation has reinitiated its phase 2 trials in 15 centers across the United States. The goal is to recruit 100 test patients and 25 control patients. A 3-year follow-up is planned.

## References

1 White G, Yu W, May J et al. Design developments and long-term results of a balloon-deployed endovascular graft (tube or bifurcated) for the repair of abdominal aortic aneurysms [abstract]. *J Endovasc Ther* 1996; 3: 82.
2 Edwards Lifesciences. *Lifepath AAA Bifurcated Graft System Manual*. Irvine, CA, 2001.
3 Wilson SE, Fujitani RM, White GH et al. Clinical experience with the Lifepath AAA endovascular graft for repair of abdominal aortic aneurysms. In: Veith FJ, ed. *Veith Symposium*. New York, 2001.

# CHAPTER 15

# Talent LPS endoluminal stent graft

Sherry D. Scovell, MD, Lisa Jordan, MSE, Roy K. Greenberg, MD

## Introduction

The first Talent stent graft (Medtronic, Inc., Minneapolis, MN) was placed for exclusion of an infrarenal abdominal aortic aneurysm (AAA) in December 1995. Since then, more than 10 000 Talent stent grafts have been placed in both the abdominal aorta (90%) and the thoracic aorta (10%) worldwide. Currently, Talent stent grafts are used in US clinical trials and are commercially available outside the United States. This chapter focuses on the Talent LPS (low-profile system) AAA stent graft (the most recent Talent design), including its design features and delivery systems, and the results from US and European clinical trials.

## Talent LPS AAA stent graft

The Talent LPS endoluminal stent graft is a modular system available in bifurcated or aorto-uni-iliac configurations (Figure 15.1). A unique feature and the greatest advantage of the Talent stent graft is the availability of customized prostheses to better accommodate each patient's anatomical variation. The device may be designed using various diameters, lengths, and tapering configurations. Also offered are various stock catalog sizes and configurations. Straight grafts are available in diameters ranging from 8 to 46 mm in increments of 2 mm, and in lengths ranging from 50 to 200 mm in increments of 10 mm. The dimensions of the bifurcated grafts are customized by choosing various combinations of body and limb diameters. Different spring configurations are available: (1) "Open Web," in which fabric is affixed to the stent at each apex, precisely following the stent pattern (Figure 15.2), and (2) stent grafts with uncovered proximal stents that have a support spring ("FreeFlo").

Most commonly, the graft is designed with a proximal uncovered stent, allowing for transrenal fixation. This may be particularly useful for an AAA with a short proximal neck, providing a means to fixate the graft in a region of the aorta that is potentially more stable than the infrarenal segment without adversely affecting renal artery patency.

The Talent stent graft, similar to most endovascular AAA devices, has four main components: (1) the support frame, which provides fixation in the artery and maintains the geometric configuration of the graft, (2) the fabric

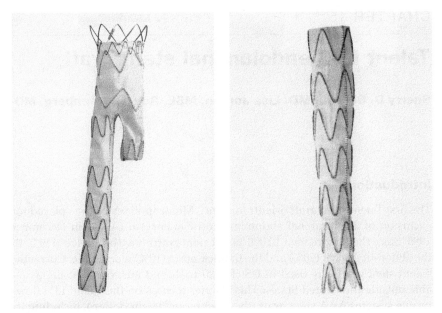

**Figure 15.1** Design configurations of the Talent LPS endoluminal stent graft (Medtronic, Inc.). Left, bifurcated; right, aorto-uni-iliac.

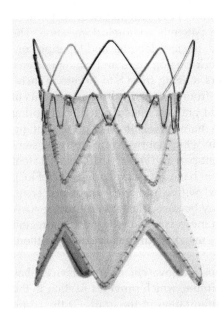

**Figure 15.2** Open Web configuration of the Talent stent graft (Medtronic, Inc.).

covering, which excludes the aneurysmal segment of the aorta from blood flow, (3) radiopaque markers, which aid in fluoroscopic visualization, and (4) sutures, which secure the components together.

## Support frame

### Stents

The support frame uses serpentine nitinol spring stents designed to provide radial pressure against the vessel wall (Figure 15.3). The springs are made of 0.02-inch-diameter round wire that has an oxide coating (titanium dioxide) to resist corrosion and improve radiopacity. The use of stents with oversized diameters ensures that adequate radial pressure will maintain the position and the seal when the stent graft is implanted. Individual stent height is approximately 15 mm. In addition to the main stents, a shorter support spring of thinner wire is affixed to the proximal end of grafts that have diameters >20 mm. This support spring decreases the likelihood of fabric infolding that may occur because of graft oversizing. Stent grafts with uncovered proximal stents and a support spring are referred to as "FreeFlo," whereas grafts with uncovered proximal stents and no support spring are designated "Bare Spring."

### Connecting bar

Nitinol connecting bars provide longitudinal support along the entire length of each graft segment. They are integral to the springs, creating a support structure for fixation in the artery and a frame to which the graft fabric is secured. The connecting bar was designed to serve three purposes: (1) to resist twisting or buckling of the graft, (2) to eliminate foreshortening by maintain-

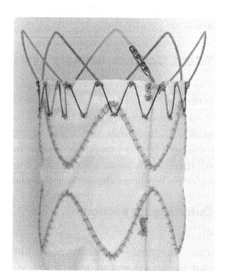

**Figure 15.3** Talent stent graft (Medtronic, Inc.), illustrating nitinol springs.

ing a fixed length, and (3) with proper orientation, to straighten anatomical curvature, thus potentially preventing kinking in tortuous vessels. For proper orientation, the connecting bar must be positioned along the greater portion of the curve (i.e., the larger or outer radius). Additionally, the connecting bar most likely provides some columnar support. Tube grafts have at least one connecting bar, and bifurcated grafts have at least two.

### Fabric covering

The Talent LPS graft material is a woven monofilament (polyethylene tereph-thalate or PET) approximately 0.09 mm thick. During *in vitro* testing, this material has had better tensile strength and wear resistance than many other fabrics. The twill square weave of the monofilament creates a highly orga-nized structure that is tightly controlled to maintain consistency, eliminate imperfections, and decrease the likelihood of fabric tears, degradation, and late dilation [1].

### Radiopaque markers

The figure-eight platinum radiopaque markers are sewn to the device to iden-tify the proximal and distal edges of the fabric and to ensure adequate overlap for modular junctions and proper placement of the proximal graft material with respect to the renal arteries. When viewed from an anteroposterior per-spective, the distribution of the markers resembles an "8," but when viewed from a lateral perspective, the markers are aligned in a straight line.

### Sutures

Each stent ring is sewn individually to the graft fabric by inlaying the stent into the fabric and suturing it securely in place using braided polyester sur-gical suture. The stents are completely sutured to minimize any micromove-ment of the stent relative to the graft material during the implant's service life, thus greatly reducing the possibility of fabric or suture wear.

### Talent CoilTrac delivery system

The most recent version of the Talent endoluminal stent graft delivery system is the CoilTrac, which is one of the simplest to use (Figure 15.4). The delivery system has three main sections: (1) the outer sheath used to constrain the stent graft, (2) the push rod used to provide positioning stability, and (3) the catheter used to provide a guidewire lumen for advancement of the system. All three sections may be secured together as a single unit or released to move independently, as desired by the user.

### Outer sheath section

#### Sheath
The stent graft is constrained within the delivery system by a polytef sheath that has an outer diameter of 18–24F, depending on the diameter, length, and

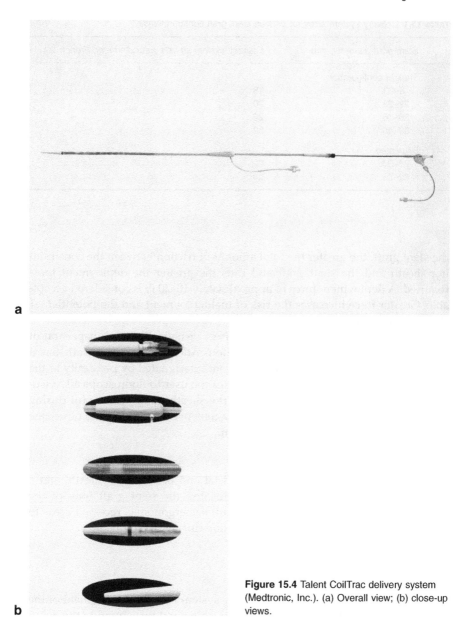

a

b

**Figure 15.4** Talent CoilTrac delivery system (Medtronic, Inc.). (a) Overall view; (b) close-up views.

configuration of the stent graft. Delivery system sizes are based on stent graft diameter and configuration (Table 15.1). These delivery system sizes are applicable for stent grafts up to 120 mm in length; stent grafts longer than 120 mm may be loaded in larger sheaths. The reason that larger delivery sheaths are used with longer stent grafts is ease of deployment—the longer

**Table 15.1** Delivery system sizes for various stent graft configurations.

| Stent graft diameter, mm | Delivery system sheath outer diameter, French |
|---|---|
| Straight configuration | |
| 8–20 | 18 |
| 22–28 | 20 |
| 30–36 | 22 |
| 38–46 | 24 |
| Bifurcated | |
| 22–30 | 22 |
| 32–36 | 24 |

the stent graft, the greater the total amount of friction between the constraining sheath and the stent graft and thus the greater the deployment force required. A deployment force of approximately 10–20 lb is considered acceptable. Greater force increases the risk of maldeployment and the potential for sheath deformation (stretching).

The sheath is translucent, allowing direct visualization and inspection of the stent graft orientation before insertion. Additionally, the sheath has a radiopaque marker band at its proximal end (designated by proximity to the heart, not to the user). This feature enables the user to fluoroscopically visualize the precise location of the end of the sheath, which is helpful during stent graft deployment and during reengagement of the sheath and nose cone before withdrawal of the delivery system.

### Sheath hub
A plastic sheath hub is affixed to the distal end of the outer sheath, and a two-way stopcock acts as a port for flushing the stent graft (one of the recommended preparation steps). The hub has ergonomic, recessed areas to facilitate handling and maintaining position during deployment.

### Push rod section

### Coil rod and plunger
A unique feature of the CoilTrac delivery system is the coiled segment of the push rod. The stainless steel coil aids in tracking and maneuvering the delivery system. The coil occupies space within the sheath, providing support and preventing the sheath from collapsing or kinking in tortuous vessels. It also provides a smooth, flexible transition between the stiffer push rod and the more flexible stent graft, eliminating a possible kink point in the system.

Just proximal to the coil is the plastic cup plunger section of the delivery system, which is recessed slightly to constrain the apexes of the distal stent graft spring. The cup plunger holds the stent graft in place during deployment and constrains the distal graft spring, reducing the likelihood of it becoming lodged between the push rod and the sheath.

### Push rod and handle

"Push rod" is a misnomer because the purpose of the push rod is to provide stability, and thus it must remain stationary during deployment. Affixed to the proximal end of the push rod are the coil and plunger described above. The rod has a handle fitted with a Touhy Borst valve on the distal end to secure the internal catheter and maintain hemostasis. The valve may be loosened to permit motion (advancement or retraction) of the internal catheter independently of the other sections of the delivery system. This independent motion is helpful when ballooning.

## Catheter section

### Flexible tip/nose cone

The proximal end of the delivery system has a tapered tip, similar to a short dilator. This tip allows for tracking, advancement, and manipulation through the access vessels, which are often tortuous, minimally compliant, and calcified. The tapered dilator tip is made of polyurethane: the proximal end is soft at the tip to facilitate navigation and the distal end is stiff to provide a good seal with the proximal end of the sheath. Caution must be exercised, however, when introducing this device into calcific or tortuous vessels. When there is an anatomical mismatch between the delivery system and the iliac arteries we liberally use conduits sewn to the common iliac artery to facilitate delivery.

### Balloon catheter

The stent graft is constrained over a multilumen catheter: one lumen is compatible with a 0.035-inch guidewire for advancement of the delivery system over a wire, and a second lumen is for inflation and deflation of the balloon. This compliant balloon is mounted on the proximal end of the catheter, just distal to the nose cone, and is made of polyurethane. It is available in various sizes depending on the stent graft size. The balloon may be used to mold the stent graft after deployment or to further expand the device in calcified arteries when sealing has not been achieved on initial deployment. There is also a stainless steel "bullet" mounted on the catheter, distal to the balloon and proximal to the stent graft, to reduce the likelihood of kinking proximal to the stent graft, which could potentially hinder or even prohibit deployment.

Also supplied with the delivery system is an inflation syringe intended for use with the balloon; however, a balloon inflator or Luer-Lok syringe may be used. (The balloon is not pressure rated; thus, inflation with a high-pressure inflator is not advised. If a high-pressure inflator is used, inflation must be performed with caution.)

## Clinical results

### US clinical trials
Clinical trials have been conducted in the United States with the Talent AAA stent graft. These phase 1 and phase 2 trials were used to determine the safety and efficacy of this specific stent graft in the treatment of infrarenal aortic aneurysms [2]. The results of the US phase 1 and phase 2 clinical trials have been published, including the technical results and the 30-day clinical outcomes. The phase 1 feasibility study was completed at six institutions to demonstrate the safety of the device and procedure. The phase 2 trial involved 17 investigational sites. Phase 1 and phase 2 trials included both a high physiologic risk group and a low physiologic risk group that were evaluated separately. In the low-risk group, endovascular repair was compared with standard open operation [3].

In the phase 1 and phase 2 trials, deployment success was defined as the ability to deliver the stent graft device into the intended position. Technical success was defined as successful deployment without endoleak at the conclusion of the procedure. All patients underwent both abdominal radiography and contrast-enhanced computed tomography after the procedure and before hospital dismissal. The patients were evaluated at 1 month, 6 months, and 1 year and then yearly.

### Phase 1 high-risk patients
The phase 1 high-risk group included 25 patients (24 males and 1 female) from six centers. The mean (± SD) aneurysm size was 61 ± 15 mm. Of these patients, 48% (12 of 25) had severe coronary artery disease, and 20% (5 of 25) had an ejection fraction of <30%. The stent grafts were successfully deployed in 92% of the patients (23 of 25). The two failed deployments were caused by difficulty with the access or delivery system, and both resulted in immediate conversion to open repair. Among the 23 successful deployments, there were seven early endoleaks, yielding a technical success rate of 78% (18 of 23 patients). The one perioperative death occurred in a patient who required conversion to open operation. During the 30-day postoperative period, two additional patients died, yielding an overall 30-day mortality of 12%. Within this follow-up period, other adverse events occurred in 40% of the patients, including limb ischemia, myocardial infarction, congestive heart failure, renal failure, and wound infection.

### Phase 2 high-risk patients
The phase 2 high-risk group included 127 patients from 17 centers. The mean (± SD) aneurysm size was 57 ± 10 mm. All patients in this group were high risk; 10% (13 of 127 patients) were older than 90 years and 15% (19 of 127 patients) had an ejection fraction of <20%. The bifurcated Talent endograft was used in 78% of the patients (99 of 127); the remainder received an aorto-uni-iliac device in conjunction with a femorofemoral artery bypass graft.

Deployment was successful in 94% of the patients (119 of 127), with an initial technical success rate of 86% (102 of 119 patients). Adverse events were infrequent, the most common complications being renal failure, congestive heart failure, and graft limb thrombosis. Additionally, the 30-day mortality rate was 1.5%.

## Phase 2 low-risk patients

Initially, the phase 2 low-risk group included 151 patients who received the first-generation Talent stent graft and delivery system. Successful deployment was achieved in 97% of the patients (147 of 151), with the remaining 3% (four patients) requiring conversion to open operation. Initial technical success was realized in 88% of the patients (130 of 147). Adverse events were noted in 20% of the patients (29 of 142) and included dissection in seven patients, renal failure in six, myocardial infarction in five, arrhythmia in three, pulmonary complications in three, and lower limb ischemia in two. Four patients required conversion. Three patients died during the 30-day follow-up period: two died of pulmonary complications and one died of a myocardial infarction.

When the Talent endograft was revised into the LPS version, the trial was modified and resubmitted under a separate investigational device exemption. A second phase 2 low-risk patient group was evaluated separately. This group consisted of 240 patients. Deployment was successful in 99% of the patients (237 of 240). Thirty-day mortality of 0.8% for the stent graft patients has been reported [3].

## EUROSTAR registry

The European Collaborators on Stent-Graft Techniques for Abdominal Aortic Aneurysm Repair (EUROSTAR) registry was initiated in 1996 to collect multicenter data on the results of endoluminal AAA repair in Europe. As of January 2001, 98 centers had reported operative data on 3264 patients. Another 149 patients were enrolled as well but had not received treatment for their aneurysms. The EUROSTAR registry covers all major endovascular AAA stent grafts, including AneuRx (Medtronic, Inc.), Ancure (Guidant Corp., Menlo Park, CA), Excluder (W.L. Gore and Associates, Inc., Flagstaff, AZ), Stentor (Boston Scientific Corp., Natick, MA), Vanguard (Boston Scientific Corp.), and Talent. Follow-up data for up to 60 months were available for these patients [4] (EUROSTAR Data Registry Centre Progress Report. January 2001).

The Talent implant data were analyzed from October 1996 to April 2000 (Talent Report. EUROSTAR Data Registry Centre. May 2000). During this time, 339 patients at 30 centers throughout Europe received a Talent AAA stent graft (either the Talent or the Talent LPS device). The mean age of the patients was 69.5 years (range, 45–92 years). The majority were categorized in American Society of Anesthesiologists (ASA) class II; however, approximately 8% of the patients were categorized in ASA class IV, which was a relative contraindication to open AAA repair. Approximately 3% of the patients were unfit to undergo general anesthesia. Hypertension and a history of smoking were the most frequent Society for Vascular Surgery/International Society for Cardiovascular Surgery risk factors, along with cardiac disease, as expected.

The mean maximal aneurysm diameter was 5.72 cm (range, 2.6–10.0 cm). The patients with a maximal aneurysm diameter of <4.0 cm had coexistent common iliac artery aneurysms that were the main indication for repair. The mean diameter of the proximal neck was 2.4 cm (range, 1.0–3.5 cm), which demonstrates that the Talent endograft may be custom-designed and ordered in various sizes, increasing the number of patients suitable for endograft repair. Nineteen patients underwent preoperative or intraoperative embolization of an inferior mesenteric artery, a hypogastric artery, or a lumbar artery. Coexisting hypogastric artery aneurysms were present in 2% of the patients.

Most of the patients (84%) underwent endoluminal repair under general anesthesia; regional or local anesthesia was used in only 16% of the patients. The mean duration of the procedure was 135.8 min (range, 12–410 min). Percutaneous transluminal angioplasty with or without stenting was the most common adjunct procedure performed at the time of Talent stent graft placement; it was performed in 8% of the patients. All patients underwent completion angiography, which showed type I endoleak as the most common type of endoleak after device deployment (present acutely in 7.5% of the patients). Device-related complications occurred in 6.6% of the patients. Acute conversion to open surgery was necessary in 2.4% of the patients.

The mean postoperative length of stay was 7 days (range, 0–70 days). Overall, there were 76 perioperative systemic complications. The most prevalent type of complication before hospital dismissal was cardiac, which occurred in 16 patients. Procedure-related complications occurred in 11 patients, six of whom required subsequent procedures before hospital dismissal. Local access site problems, such as bleeding, hematoma, arterial thrombosis, and peripheral emboli, occurred in 9.6% of the patients.

A total of 214 patients who received the Talent device were available for 30-day follow-up. Endoleaks were present in 15 patients at this time (five proximal, five distal, and five midgraft). Migration was noted in two patients. Five additional interventions were required in the first month after hospital dismissal. These 30-day data were similar to the EUROSTAR registry data as a whole. The 30-day results were also similar between patients who received the Talent device and patients in the overall registry, respectively, for endoleak rate (7% vs 6.5%), migration rate (0.9% vs 0.3%), and subsequent intervention rate (2.3% vs 2.6%).

Based on the data available at the time of manuscript preparation, the 1-year freedom from death rate was 93.2% in the Talent group and 91.3% in the registry. Freedom from persistent endoleak was 95.1% in the Talent group and 90.7% in the registry. Freedom from secondary intervention was 88.6% in the

Talent group and 84.7% in the registry (Talent Report, EUROSTAR Data Registry Centre, May 2000).

## Conclusions

The Talent stent graft can be used to treat aneurysms with neck diameters larger than 28 mm, unlike the other endografts currently available in the United States. It may be customized to individual specifications, and the element of suprarenal fixation extends the number of aneurysms that may be treated with this graft. Technically, the deployment system is one of the easiest to use and deployment success is relatively high, based on the latest US trial. With the introduction of the Talent LPS, the rate of adverse events has decreased. Similarly, the data from the Talent EUROSTAR registry compare favorably with the overall registry data.

## References

1  Criado FJ, Wilson EP, Wellons E, Abul-Khoudoud O, Gnanasekeram H. Early experience with the Talent stent-graft system for endoluminal repair of abdominal aortic aneurysms. *Tex Heart Inst J* 2000; **27**: 128–35.
2  Criado FJ, Fry PD, Machan LS, Twena M, Patten P. The Talent endoluminal AAA stent-graft system: report of the phase I USA trial, and summary of worldwide experience. *J Mal Vasc* 1998; **23**: 371–3.
3  Criado FJ, Fairman RM, Becker GJ, Talent LPS Pivotal Clinical Trial Investigators. Talent LPS AAA stent graft: results of a pivotal clinical trial. *J Vasc Surg* 2003; **37**: 709–15.
4  Laheij RJ, van Marrewijk CJ, for the EUROSTAR Group. The evolving technique of endovascular stenting of abdominal aortic aneurysm: time for reappraisal. *Eur J Vasc Endovasc Surg* 2001; **22**: 436–42.

# CHAPTER 16

# Balloon-expandable stent and polytef-based endograft for repair of complex and ruptured abdominal aortic aneurysms

**Takao Ohki, MD, Frank J. Veith, MD**

## Introduction

To improve on the shortcomings of surgical repair of abdominal aortic aneurysms (AAAs), transluminally placed endovascular graft (EVG) repair has emerged as a potential alternative [1]. EVG repair can be performed through small incisions in the groin, leading to less postoperative discomfort, shorter length of hospital stay, and faster recovery. In addition, EVGs can be used to treat patients who are not surgical candidates because they have comorbid conditions.

EVG repair is not a panacea, however, and it has several limitations, including poorer durability than surgical repair. Another weakness of EVG repair is that it may not be applicable to the majority of patients with AAAs because it requires that AAAs meet certain anatomical criteria [2–5]. Common anatomical characteristics that exclude the use of an EVG include (1) an iliac artery that is inadequate for the introduction of the EVG, (2) a short and wide proximal aortic neck, (3) an angulated or irregular proximal aortic neck, and (4) coexisting bilateral common iliac artery aneurysms. The reasons for some of these exclusion criteria are that all currently available EVGs use a self-expanding stent and that the delivery system is relatively stiff and large. In addition, the use of an EVG requires precise and often time-consuming preoperative measurements, so a ruptured AAA requiring urgent repair is not a candidate for EVG repair. Because of these limiting factors, various authors have estimated that only 30–50% of all AAAs may be treated endovascularly.

To overcome these limitations, as well as to treat patients with ruptured AAAs, we have developed an EVG that uses a balloon-expandable stent that was first introduced by Parodi *et al.* [1]. This chapter describes the value and limitations of a balloon-expandable stent and polytef-based EVG (Figure 16.1a,b)

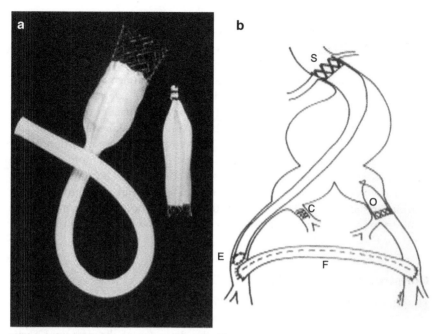

**Figure 16.1** (a) Montefiore endovascular graft (MEG) and the occluder device. (b) Drawing of a complex aneurysm repair using the MEG. The cranial end of the MEG is fixed within the proximal neck with a large Palmaz stent (S) (Cordis Corp.). In this example, the bare portion of the stent is deployed across the orifice of the renal arteries. The distal end of the endovascular graft is secured to the femoral artery by a hand-sewn endoluminal anastomosis (E). The occluder device (O) is deployed in the contralateral common iliac artery to preserve at least one internal iliac artery. C, embolization coils; F, femorofemoral bypass.

## Development of the Montefiore endovascular graft

The Montefiore endovascular graft (MEG) was derived from the Parodi graft, which was fabricated from a Palmaz stent (Cordis Corp., Miami, FL) and a Dacron graft (DuPont, Wilmington, DE) [1]. The most significant advantage of this device is that it uses a balloon-expandable stent that has the highest radial force of any stent used in other EVGs. This allows one to treat an AAA that has a short and angulated proximal aortic neck without subjecting the native artery to continued expansion, as occurs with other EVGs.

The current MEG has resulted from several modifications that have increased its versatility and ease of use [6,7]. For example, it uses a polytef graft instead of a Dacron graft (Figure 16.1a). Previously, it was necessary to accurately measure the length of the graft preoperatively so that the distal end could be fixed in the common iliac artery or the external iliac artery by a second stent. A precise measurement was often difficult to make, adding complexity to the procedure. The current MEG graft is made long enough so that in each case the distal end of the graft emerges from the insertion site in the femoral artery. The graft is cut to the appropriate length as it emerges from the artery and is anastomosed within the femoral artery. This greatly enhances the ease of the procedure, eliminating the preoperative length measurement and a potential endoleak site at the distal attachment site. In addition, because the EVG covers the inside of the entire external and common iliac arteries, dissection of the external iliac artery (which occurs often with insertion of an introducer sheath) can be repaired simultaneously.

Another modification was placement of the proximal bare portion of the stent proximal to the orifice of the renal artery. This provides more secure fixation of the proximal stent even in cases with aortic necks shorter than 1.0 cm. For the delivery system, we were able to decrease the outside diameter of the introducer sheath from 24F to 18F or 20F. All these modifications, along with some technical modifications, allowed us to expand the anatomical indications for EVG repairs.

## Construction of the MEG

The MEG device is constructed from 6-mm polytef grafts (Bard Peripheral Vascular, Inc., Tempe, AZ) [6,7]. The proximal 4-cm portion of each graft is expanded to 30 mm to accommodate the diameter of the proximal aortic neck (Figure 16.2a,b). The remainder of the graft is dilated up to 10 mm.

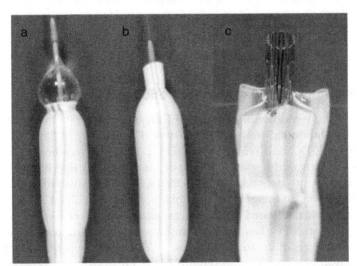

**Figure 16.2** Dilatation of the polytef graft. (a) If the dilatation balloon is not completely inserted within the polytef graft, it will lead to uneven dilatation. (b) The polytef graft should cover both ends of the balloon. (c) The dilated polytef graft is sewn to the Palmaz stent (Cordis Corp.) using eight "U" stitches placed at 12, 3, 6, and 9 o'clock (two stitches at every quarter). A gold marker denotes the cranial end of the endograft.

Expansion is accomplished by a gradual dilation with percutaneous translu-minal angioplasty balloons and an esophageal dilatation balloon (Boston Sci-entific Corp., Natick, MA). It is important to place the dilatation balloon well within the polytef graft to facilitate uniform stretching of the polytef and to prevent tearing. The graft is then sutured to a Palmaz stent (P-4014 or P-5014; Cordis Corp.) with eight "U" stitches so as to overlap one-half the length of the stent (Figure 16.2c). Four metallic markers are sutured to the proximal end of the graft material so that the end of the polytef covering can be visualized fluoroscopically. The stent graft is then crimped onto a 25-mm balloon (Maxi LD; Cordis Corp.) and loaded into a 16F sheath (Cook, Inc., Bloomington, IN). This balloon can be dilated up to 27 mm.

The occluder device, which is placed in the contralateral iliac artery to prevent retrograde filling of the aneurysm, is also made from polytef and a Palmaz stent (Figure 16.1a). Two ligatures are used to occlude one end of the polytef graft. A Palmaz stent (P-4014 or P-308) is attached to the other end of the polytef graft by means of four "U" stitches. The occluder device is loaded onto an angioplasty balloon (12–20 mm, Opta or Maxi LD; Cordis Corp.) and then inserted into either a 14F or a 16F sheath, depending on the size of the balloon.

## Operative and adjunctive techniques

### Coil embolization of the hypogastric artery

Coil embolization of the hypogastric artery ipsilateral to the graft insertion site is carried out if the distal landing zone is distal to the orifice of the inter-nal iliac artery. Coil embolization (Gianturco coils; Cook, Inc.) is usually per-formed at the time of EVG insertion in the operating room, although it can be performed preoperatively. Coil embolization has been performed routinely with all MEG aorto-uni-femoral grafts.

### Deployment of the EVG

An Amplatz Super-Stiff guidewire (Cook, Inc.) is inserted into the thoracic aorta, and the 16F sheath containing the MEG is then advanced over the wire. After the location of the most distal renal artery is confirmed, the outer sheath is retracted and the proximal stent is deployed by inflating the balloon. The cephalad end of the graft material in the MEG has a metallic marker for fluoroscopic visualization. The graft is deployed so that this marker is placed just distal to the most distal renal artery. The bare stent above the marker usually covers the orifice of the renal arteries. The balloon is semicompliant, and its size can be modified by simply changing its inflation pressure (Figure 16.3). The balloon is generally sized 1 mm larger than the aortic neck diam-eter, which is measured from the preoperative computed tomographic scan and intraoperative angiogram.

After the main EVG is deployed, the introducer sheath and the deployment balloon are retrieved. The endograft is long enough so that the distal end

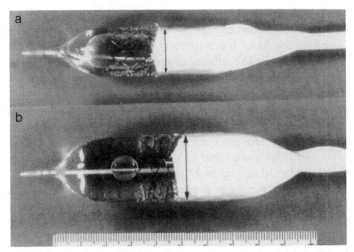

**Figure 16.3** The proximal stent is fitted to various aortic neck diameters by changing the inflation pressure of the deployment balloon. (a) When the balloon is inflated to 2 atm (202 kPA), the proximal stent is expanded to 20 mm (arrow). (b) When the balloon is inflated to 6 atm (606 kPA), the stent is expanded to 28 mm (arrow). (Reprinted from Ohki T, Veith FJ, Endovascular grafts and other image-guided catheter-based adjuncts to improve the treatment of ruptured aortoiliac aneurysms, *Ann Surg* 2000; **232**: 466–79, Copyright 2000, with permission from Lippincott, Williams and Wilkins.)

emerges from the femoral arteriotomy site. A 9F sheath is then inserted into the distal end of the graft. Balloon angioplasty is performed throughout the entire length of the graft to ensure its full expansion and to eliminate any possible compression of the graft. A SMART stent (8 × 80 mm; Cordis Corp.) is usually placed in the common and external iliac arteries.

## Management of the distal anastomosis

If the distal end of the graft terminates in the common femoral artery, an endovascular anastomosis is performed. A surgical clamp is placed proximally to the arteriotomy site and the endograft is cut to the appropriate length as it emerges from the femoral artery (Figure 16.4a). A running suture of 5–0 polypropylene is used to securely attach the distal end to the native artery (Figure 16.4b).

If an aorto-uni-iliac graft is used, the distal end is secured by a second Palmaz stent. The distal end of the endograft can be visualized radiologically if a metallic marker has been sutured in the end. A loop suture may be useful to prevent migration of the distal end of the graft into the aneurysm when one passes the second stent into the graft before its deployment.

## Deployment of the occluder device

After deployment of the aorto-uni-femoral EVG, an occluder device is placed in the contralateral common iliac artery. Placement of a standard

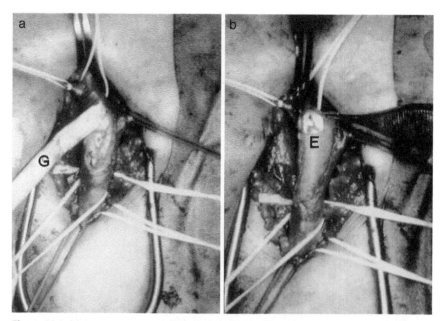

**Figure 16.4** (a) The distal end (G) of the uncut endovascular graft (EVG) emerges from the femoral arteriotomy site. (b) After the EVG is cut to the appropriate length by trimming the distal end, a hand-sewn endoluminal anastomosis (E) is performed within the femoral artery. The arteriotomy site becomes the anastomosis site for the subsequent femorofemoral bypass. (Reprinted from Ohki T, Veith FJ, Endovascular grafts and other image-guided catheter-based adjuncts to improve the treatment of ruptured aortoiliac aneurysms, *Ann Surg* 2000; **232**: 466–79, Copyright 2000, with permission from Lippincott, Williams and Wilkins.)

femorofemoral bypass using a ringed polytef graft completes the procedure (Figure 16.1b).

Completion arteriography and pressure gradient studies are performed to assure technical adequacy and the absence of an endoleak. If an endoleak is present because of too distal deployment of the proximal stent, a polytef-covered Palmaz stent is deployed proximally to the previously deployed graft to seal the leak. If an endoleak is present because of underdeployment of the stent, further dilation of the proximal stent is usually sufficient to seal the leak.

## Inclusion criteria for the MEG

We have chosen to use commercial devices and open surgical repair before the MEG whenever possible. Thus, we used the MEG only for patients who could not be treated with commercial devices or with open surgical repair (Figure 16.5a,b). Patients were most often excluded from use of commercial EVGs because of severe angulation of the proximal aortic neck, a short proximal aortic neck, or small and diseased iliac arteries. Generally, we would

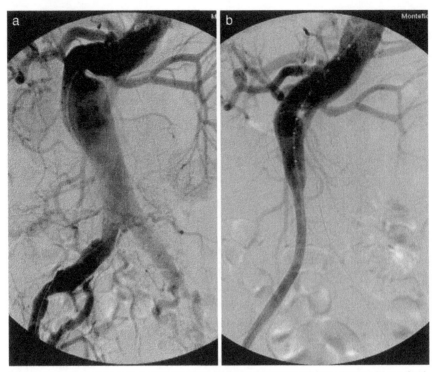

**Figure 16.5** (a) An anatomically complex abdominal aortic aneurysm. Note the severe proximal aortic neck angulation (110°) as well as the occluded left external iliac artery. (b) Completion angiogram after Montefiore endovascular graft repair. Because of the strong radial force of the Palmaz stent (Cordis Corp.), an excellent seal was achieved despite the severe neck angulation.

not treat a patient with the MEG if the patient had bilateral long iliac artery occlusions or a proximal aortic neck shorter than 5 mm or wider than 28 mm.

## Current clinical experience with the MEG

At Montefiore Medical Center, between 1997 and 2002, 82 patients were treated with the MEG; they had nonruptured, anatomically complex AAAs and they were not good candidates for commercial devices or open surgical repair [8]. By virtue of the inclusion criteria, patients who received the MEG were older and had more severe comorbid conditions than patients treated with commercial EVGs. Vascular surgeons referred 34% of these patients. Patients were excluded from treatment with commercial EVG protocols or treatment with open surgical repair for the following reasons: short proximal (<1.0 cm) or angulated (>60°) aortic neck ($n = 46$); the lack of an acceptable distal landing zone because of enlarged or aneurysmal common iliac arteries ($n$ = 12); small diameter or tortuous iliac arteries or iliac arteries with extensive occlusive disease ($n$ = 21); and a small distal aorta that could not accommodate a bifurcated graft ($n$ = 3).

The 30-day operative mortality rate was 7.3%, and the technical success rate with successful delivery and absence of an endoleak was 99%. In one patient, a proximal type I endoleak could not be treated. A covered stent was placed but failed to seal the leak. Because this patient had various comorbid conditions in addition to a history of an aborted attempt at open repair, further attempts to treat the leak were terminated. Although various complications occurred after MEG repair, none required conversion to open repair.

During a mean follow-up period of 35 months, only one other patient had a type I endoleak. This patient returned 18 months postoperatively, after a proximal type I endoleak developed. The cause of the endoleak was distal deployment of the MEG. This patient was treated by deploying a second MEG within the previous one.

Four MEGs thrombosed during the follow-up period and were treated with axillobifemoral bypass (three patients) or thrombectomy (one patient). One patient required a below-knee amputation because of MEG thrombosis. Two additional patients underwent stent placement for stenosis within the MEG limb. At 35 months, the overall freedom from failure rate was 94%. Two patients underwent open conversion for the treatment of endotension; absence of an endoleak was confirmed during open repair. Overall, freedom from any secondary intervention was 89% and freedom from open conversion was 97%.

## Long-term outcome with the Parodi EVG

Parodi has been using a similar balloon-expandable stent graft since 1990 and has reported the long-term follow-up results (JC Parodi, pers. comm., July 23, 2001). One disadvantage of using a self-expandable stent is the frequent occurrence of proximal aortic neck dilatation. Parodi specifically examined the change in proximal aortic neck diameter. He used computed tomography to compare the neck diameter before treatment with the neck diameter at 5 years and later in 30 patients (Figures 16.6 and 16.7). Because the balloon-expandable stent does not exert ongoing force to the aortic wall, no enlargement of the proximal neck was observed. This is an important advantage of the balloon-expandable stent in addition to the other aspects described above.

## Use of the MEG for ruptured AAAs

### Limitations of surgical repair of ruptured AAAs

Since the 1960s, when the first successful repair of an infrarenal AAA was reported, several important advances have been made in the nonsurgical aspects of care. These include transportation of patients, their critical care, the

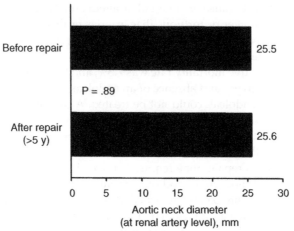

**Figure 16.6** Aortic neck diameter at the level of the renal artery before Parodi endograft repair and at a mean follow-up of 7.5 years (*n* = 30). (Courtesy of Juan Parodi.)

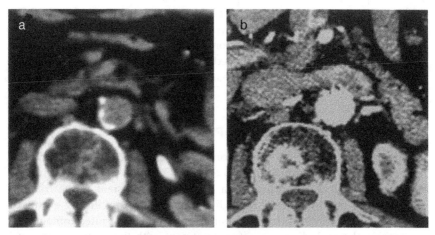

**Figure 16.7** (a) Preoperative computed tomographic (CT) scan shows the proximal aortic neck diameter measuring 25 mm (September 1990). (b) Seven-year follow-up CT scan shows the proximal aortic neck diameter remaining stable at 25 mm (May 1997). (Courtesy of Juan Parodi.)

management of their cardiac dysfunction, and pharmacologic support. In spite of these efforts, operative mortality rates have not improved significantly and still range from 24% to 70% [9,10]. In part, this is because the basic surgical techniques for repairing ruptured AAAs have changed little, although a number of minor improvements have been introduced. These minor improvements include supraceliac clamping, suturing the graft within the aneurysm without excising it, more frequent use of tube grafts, and use of prostheses with less porosity. General anesthesia, laparotomy techniques, the need for extensive dissection, and the accompanying invasiveness and blood loss in open repair have, however, remained largely unchanged and may be responsible for the poor outcome.

## Inherent limitations and potential benefits of endovascular graft repair for ruptured AAAs

Although EVGs are theoretically appealing because of their minimally invasive nature, their use in the treatment of ruptured AAAs or iliac artery aneurysms has been limited [11,12]. One important reason has been the need for preoperative anatomical measurements of the aneurysm and adjacent arteries so that an appropriate size and configuration of graft can be selected. The resulting delay has been deemed inappropriate in the urgency of ruptured AAAs. In addition, inserting an endograft and completing the endovascular repair may be time consuming, resulting in further delay for gaining control at the aorta proximal to the aneurysm and achieving hemodynamic stability. We have used the "one-size-fits-most" MEG as well as transbrachially placed occlusion balloons to overcome these inherent problems [12].

## Indications for endovascular repair of ruptured AAAs

In cases of ruptured AAA in which preoperative computed tomography or angiography have not already been performed, an aortogram is first obtained in the operating room and a decision is made on the feasibility of endovascular repair. The exclusion criteria for endovascular repair include pararenal AAAs (neck length <5 mm), proximal neck diameter >28 mm, bilateral long iliac artery occlusions, or mycotic aneurysm. Otherwise, all patients are preferentially treated with EVGs. The surgical technique for ruptured AAAs is basically the same as for elective AAAs. One modification is to perform coil embolization of the internal iliac artery after the EVG is deployed if the patient is hemodynamically unstable.

## Patients and methods

Between January 2000 and July 2001, 12 consecutive patients with ruptured AAAs were treated at our institution. All patients presented with acute onset of abdominal pain or back pain (or both) and other signs such as profound hypotension. Treatment included the features listed below.

1 As advocated by Crawford [13], minimal fluid resuscitation was used despite hypotension (hypotensive hemostasis).

2 In each case, a guidewire was inserted percutaneously into the descending aorta via the brachial artery under local anesthesia and fluoroscopic control. An aortic occlusion balloon was inserted over this wire, and control at the aorta proximal to the aneurysm was gained in six patients whose systolic blood pressure was <50 mmHg either before or during anesthesia induction.

The occlusion balloon was inserted through a 14F sheath. After control in the supraceliac portion of the aorta was gained with this balloon, the femoral arteries were exposed and an infrarenal occlusion balloon was deployed in exchange for the supraceliac balloon so as to perfuse the viscera (Figure 16.8). This balloon was used as needed in cases in which open surgery was performed.

3 Intra-operative aortography was performed. On the basis of the angiographic or computed tomographic findings, the feasibility of EVG repair was determined, and EVG repair was performed if possible.

4 The MEG graft was used if EVG repair was indicated.

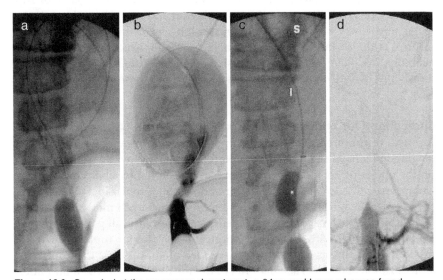

**Figure 16.8.** On arrival at the emergency department, a 64-year-old man who was found unconscious at home had a systolic blood pressure of 40 mmHg, a distended abdomen, and a pulsatile mass. With a diagnosis of presumed ruptured abdominal aortic aneurysm (AAA), the patient was taken to the operating room without a preoperative computed tomographic scan. (a) Under local anesthesia, a brachial wire and then an occlusion balloon were placed in the abdominal aorta. When the occlusion balloon was inflated in the supraceliac aorta, the systolic blood pressure increased immediately to 110 mmHg. The curvature of the brachial wire indicates a large AAA. (b) With the occlusion balloon inflated, aortography confirmed the diagnosis of an AAA. The well-defined infrarenal neck fulfilled the inclusion criteria for endovascular graft repair. Proximal occlusion and a lack of prograde flow resulted in underfilling of the visceral and renal arteries. (c) Both femoral arteries were exposed, the sheath was inserted into the abdominal aorta, and the supraceliac occlusion balloon (S) was deflated. It was exchanged for an infrarenal occlusion balloon (I) inserted from the femoral artery. (d) Aortography with the brachial catheter confirmed perfusion of the visceral and renal arteries. (Reprinted from Ohki T, Veith FJ, Endovascular grafts and other image-guided catheter-based adjuncts to improve the treatment of ruptured aortoiliac aneurysms, *Ann Surg* 2000; **232**: 466–79, Copyright 2000, with permission from Lippincott, Williams and Wilkins.)

## Results

EVG repair was performed in eight cases and standard open repair was performed in the other four cases. Technical and clinical success was achieved in 11 cases, with resolution of preoperative symptoms. One patient died of respiratory distress despite successful deployment of the MEG. Postoperative computed tomographic scans did not show an endoleak in any of the EVG-treated cases. Abdominal compartment syndrome caused by a large intra-abdominal hematoma developed in two EVG-treated cases. This resolved after the hematoma was evacuated through a limited abdominal incision (Figure 16.9).

### Theoretical advantages of EVG repair in the treatment of ruptured AAAs

#### Ability to gain control proximally before general anesthesia induction

Initially, patients with ruptured AAA may be severely hypotensive; however, in many patients, especially those who arrive at the hospital emergently,

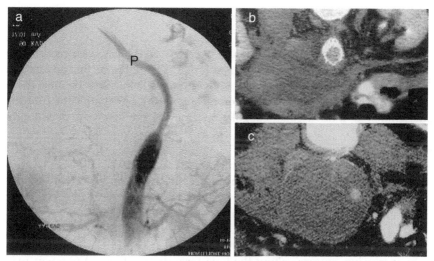

**Figure 16.9** (a) On completion angiography, the large aneurysm was completely excluded. There was no evidence of an endoleak. P, proximal Palmaz stent (Cordis Corp.). (b), (c) On postoperative contrast-enhanced computed tomography, the aneurysm was completely excluded and the contrast medium was confined within the endovascular graft. Even after hematoma evacuation for abdominal compartment syndrome, much of the hematoma remained in the retroperitoneal space. (Reprinted from Ohki T, Veith FJ, Endovascular grafts and other image-guided catheter-based adjuncts to improve the treatment of ruptured aortoiliac aneurysms, *Ann Surg* 2000; **232**: 466–79, Copyright 2000, with permission from Lippincott, Williams and Wilkins.)

blood pressure may stabilize at a nonlethal level, mainly as a result of vasoconstriction. Occasionally this vasoconstriction is released on induction of
general anesthesia. This may be partially responsible for the high mortality
rate after open repair. A guidewire and, if needed, an occlusion balloon
can be inserted into the abdominal aorta through a percutaneous puncture
under local anesthesia, however, thereby maintaining vasoconstriction. The
brachial balloon has been useful even in cases in which open surgery was
required.

### Ability to deploy the graft from a remote access site

EVGs can be inserted and deployed through a remote access site, thereby
obviating the need for laparotomy and, more importantly, eliminating the
technical difficulties encountered when performing a standard repair in this
setting. The retroperitoneal structures are often automatically distorted and
obscured because of a large hematoma. This may lead not only to technical
difficulties but also to inadvertent injury of the inferior vena cava, the left
renal vein or its genital branches, the duodenum, the ureters, and other
surrounding structures. These iatrogenic injuries have been the cause of
significant operative mortality and morbidity after standard surgery for
ruptured aneurysms. In contrast, EVG repair is performed within the arterial
tree, which is unaffected by the extravasated blood or previous operative
scarring.

### Less blood loss

The amount of blood loss during elective EVG repair has been reported to
be less than that accompanying open repair. The value of this advantage,
however, is far greater in patients with ruptured aneurysms because these
patients have already lost a considerable amount of blood after the rupture;
disseminated intravascular coagulation from blood loss is a devastating
complication.

### Minimizing hypothermia by eliminating laparotomy

Hypothermia from poor perfusion and laparotomy can exacerbate coagu-
lopathy, which is one of the causes of death after surgical repair. EVG repair
minimizes the extent of hypothermia by avoiding laparotomy.

### The "bridge graft" concept

The increasing concerns about the long-term durability of EVG repair may
be of less importance when EVG repair is used for ruptured AAAs. If the
patient's condition is initially stabilized with the EVG, the patient can safely
undergo an elective open repair if failure is detected or anticipated. Intui-
tively, the mortality rate for this elective conversion would be less than
for open repair at the time of rupture. Thus, we believe that there is still
significant merit in performing EVG repair even if the endograft is not
durable.

## Summary

Although the MEG may be more technically demanding to use, it has been a useful tool to treat AAAs that are not candidates for either commercial EVGs or standard surgical procedures. The chief advantages include (1) low-profile delivery system, (2) use of a balloon-expandable stent with strong radial force, (3) aorto-uni-femoral configuration, (4) "one-size-fits-most" intraoperative customization, and (5) durable outcome of up to 10 years because of a strong proximal fixation and the lack of metal-fabric interaction. Although the number of cases is small, our experience shows that EVG repair of ruptured AAAs and iliac artery aneurysms is feasible and effective. A prospective randomized trial comparing MEG repair with open surgery in the treatment of ruptured AAAs is needed to show the true value of this approach in the management of ruptured AAAs.

## References

1 Parodi JC, Palmaz JC, Barone HD. Transfemoral intraluminal graft implantation for abdominal aortic aneurysms. *Ann Vasc Surg* 1991; **5**: 491–9.
2 Balm R, Stokking R, Kaatee R *et al.* Computed tomographic angiographic imaging of abdominal aortic aneurysms: implications for transfemoral endovascular aneurysm management. *J Vasc Surg* 1997; **26**: 231–7.
3 Ohki T, Veith FJ. Patient selection for endovascular repair of abdominal aortic aneurysms: changing the threshold for intervention. *Semin Vasc Surg* 1999; **12**: 226–34.
4 Broeders IA, Blankensteijn JD. Preoperative imaging of the aortoiliac anatomy in endovascular aneurysm surgery. *Semin Vasc Surg* 1999; **12**: 306–14.
5 Sternbergh WC III, Carter G, York JW, Yoselevitz M, Money SR. Aortic neck angulation predicts adverse outcome with endovascular abdominal aortic aneurysm repair. *J Vasc Surg* 2002; **35**: 482–6.
6 Ohki T, Marin ML, Veith FJ *et al.* Endovascular aortounifemoral grafts and femorofemoral bypass for bilateral limb-threatening ischemia. *J Vasc Surg* 1996; **24**: 984–96.
7 Ohki T, Veith FJ. Minimally invasive vascular surgery. In: Brooks DC, ed. *Current Review of Minimally Invasive Surgery*, 3rd edn. Philadelphia: Current Medicine, 1998: 125–36.
8 Ohki T, Veith FJ, Shaw P *et al.* Increasing incidence of midterm and long-term complications after endovascular graft repair of abdominal aortic aneurysms: a note of caution based on a 9-year experience. *Ann Surg* 2001; **234**: 323–34.
9 Ernst CB. Abdominal aortic aneurysm. *N Engl J Med* 1993; **328**: 1167–72.
10 Noel AA, Gloviczki P, Cherry KJ Jr *et al.* Ruptured abdominal aortic aneurysms: the excessive mortality rate of conventional repair. *J Vasc Surg* 2001; **34**: 41–6.
11 Ohki T, Veith FJ. Endovascular grafts and other image-guided catheter-based adjuncts to improve the treatment of ruptured aortoiliac aneurysms. *Ann Surg* 2000; **232**: 466–79.
12 Hinchliffe RJ, Yusuf SW, Macierewicz JA *et al.* Endovascular repair of ruptured abdominal aortic aneurysm: a challenge to open repair? Results of a single center experience in 20 patients. *Eur J Vasc Endovasc Surg* 2001; **22**: 528–34.
13 Crawford ES. Ruptured abdominal aortic aneurysm. *J Vasc Surg* 1991; **13**: 348–50.

## CHAPTER 17

# Custom Dacron–stainless steel stent grafts

**Albert G. Hakaim, MD, Timothy M. Schmitt, MD**

## Introduction

Endovascular aneurysm repair (EVAR) began when several surgeons designed and deployed stent grafts constructed from Dacron (DuPont, Wilmington, DE) sewn to stainless steel stents. Since 1987, these early grafts have served as prototypes for devices currently completing phase 3 clinical trials and for devices that have received US Food and Drug Administration (FDA) approval.

While surgeons await approval of devices for treating patients who have aortas that are not anatomically suitable for the currently available stent grafts (e.g., wide or short proximal aortic necks), custom stent grafts continue to be important in EVAR for high-risk surgical patients. We have been involved in the construction and deployment of custom devices since June 1999 as part of an FDA-approved investigational device exemption (IDE G990024; A.G.H.) for high-risk surgical patients. To date, we have treated 23 patients with custom devices. Several devices were placed before FDA approval of any stent graft, and the remainder were placed in high-risk surgical patients, whose aortas anatomically precluded the use of a currently available device.

The purpose of this chapter is to provide basic elements of the history, construction, and deployment of Dacron–stainless steel devices. This information may help the reader better understand the advantages and disadvantages of endovascular devices. In addition, should the occasion arise to construct and deploy a custom graft segment, this chapter may serve as a guide.

## Historical perspective

In 1969, the concept of an endovascular prosthesis to bridge (or exclude) thoracic, abdominal aortic, and iliac aneurysms was first suggested by Dotter [1]. Subsequent human investigations were reported by Volodos and colleagues at the Kharkov Center for Cardiovascular Surgery, Kharkov, Ukraine [2]. These early stent grafts were constructed from woven Dacron sewn onto zigzag-shaped springs termed "fixing elements." These devices were introduced via the femoral artery and placed in the iliac artery in 19 patients, in the abdominal aorta in eight patients, and in the thoracic aorta in four patients.

The modern era of EVAR began 22 years later, with the report by Parodi *et al.* [3]. Their animal investigations and encouraging initial clinical results using Dacron grafts with balloon-expandable stents stimulated clinical and industrial interest in EVAR.

## Evolution of stent graft construction

Stainless steel Gianturco Z stents (Cook, Inc., Bloomington, IN) were used initially as proximally covered stents, without longitudinal stents, for Dacron grafts that were tapered to conform to the aortic and iliac diameters. Because these early devices lacked the additional bulk and support of longitudinal Z stents, the stent graft could be compressed easily, loaded, and deployed in an 18F sheath. To prevent kinking of the graft limb and subsequent thrombosis, however, placement of Wallstents within the body of the graft became routine [4–6]. Subsequent development led to a fully supported Dacron Z stent that required a larger introducer sheath but alleviated the need for placing a Wallstent [7].

Despite the proximal diameter of the stent graft being oversized by at least 10% to generate radial force, the durability of these early stent grafts was hindered by distal migration of the device [8]. The frequency of distal migration led several groups to modify stent graft construction to include a "bare" stent (that is, a stent with an uncovered proximal end) with hooks and barbs. In theory, the apposition of the bare stent to the aorta adjacent to the renal artery would lead to a more durable fixation [7–9]. However, because the struts of the bare stent traversed the renal ostia, the effect on renal blood flow and subsequent renal function became an immediate concern. During a 4-year period, though, in a series of 90 stent grafts with bare stents traversing the renal arteries, there was no significant deterioration in renal function and no documented renal artery occlusion [10].

Our current design of custom Dacron–stainless steel stent grafts incorporates an endoskeleton of Gianturco Z stents, to support the length of the graft, and a bare suprarenal stent, to allow for durable fixation. Before construction, all diameter measurements were obtained from computed tomographic scans, with and without contrast media, at a 3-mm slice thickness, as described in Chapter 3. All measurements were made from one outer wall to the other outer wall, at a point where the aortic diameter was least affected by the obliquity of the aortic neck. Length measurements were obtained using a standard calibrated angiographic catheter. In general, angiographic length measurements are more accurate than those obtained from computed tomographic scans, because angiographic measurements are not affected by aortoiliac tortuosity.

After the dimensions of the stent graft were obtained, a Verisoft Dacron graft (Meadox Medicals, Inc., Oakland, NJ) with the appropriate proximal and distal diameters, allowing for a 4- to 5-mm oversize, was spatulated to allow for a transition zone length of approximately 20 mm (Figure 17.1). This rather short transition zone reduces the bulk of the fabric, while ensuring sufficient length at the proximal end for apposition with the aortic neck.

The edges of the spatulated segments were melted with an ophthalmic cautery to prevent fraying of the fabric. The segments were sewn using 6–0 polytef suture (W.L. Gore and Associates, Inc., Flagstaff, AZ) in a continuous fashion. A new suture was started at each apex and tied at the midpoint of the suture line. Stents were placed within the spatulated graft after their restraining sutures were removed. The stents were loaded in a 12F sheath (Cook, Inc., Bloomington, IN) and released while the stent graft was transilluminated. This allowed for precise placement and orientation of the stents. A maximal gap of 3 mm was created between stents. A larger gap caused loss of axial orientation during deployment and telescoping of the device within the delivery sheath. Each islet of the stent was affixed to the stent graft using 6–0 polytef suture. For each stent graft, proximal and distal extensions were constructed routinely. These extensions were 60 mm long because this was the minimum length that allowed for coverage of two stents. In addition, an occluder for the contralateral common iliac artery was constructed. This consisted of a segment of Dacron graft with a diameter that was 4–5 mm larger than the diameter of the artery. After two Z stents were deployed and affixed, the proximal end of the occluder was oversewn with 6–0 polytef suture. All stent graft components underwent a simulated deployment through a Keller-

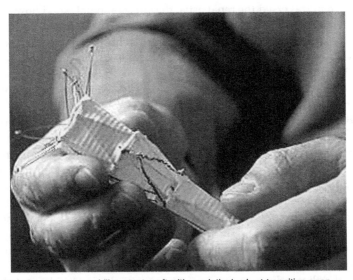

**Figure 17.1** Custom aorto-uni-iliac stent graft with a relatively short transition zone.

Timmerman sheath (Cook, Inc.) of an appropriate diameter. The components were then sterilized with ethylene oxide.

## Delivery systems

The diameter of the delivery system was selected according to the stent graft diameter and the size of the stents used in its construction. The bulk of the stent graft depended on the stent diameter. Stent diameters larger than 20 mm increase the bulk of the device. The size of the delivery sheath ranged from 20F to 24F, depending on the specific stent graft being deployed. The loading sheath was 2F smaller than the delivery sheath.

The stent graft was placed in the loading sheath by passing a stiff guidewire, which was covered with a 4F angiographic catheter, through the loading sheath (Figure 17.2). The stent graft was then "back-loaded" (that is, pulled in the reverse direction) over the angiographic catheter, with the aid of a restraining silk suture (Figure 17.3). The stiff guidewire within the loading sheath was removed, and the angiographic catheter was used to place the stent graft into the loading sheath and onto the stiff guidewire within the delivery sheath. After the stent graft was placed into the loading sheath, the tapered tip of the introducer of the loading sheath was trimmed and removed. This was necessary to avoid perforating the stent graft as it was advanced into the delivery sheath. At the time of deployment, the angiographic catheter was withdrawn before the loading sheath introducer was passed. After the stent graft was within the delivery sheath, the loading sheath

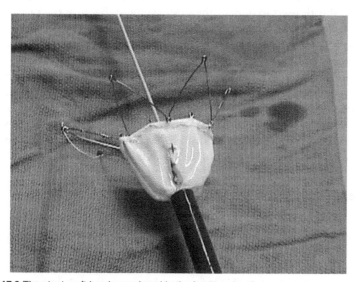

**Figure 17.2** The stent graft has been placed in the loading sheath.

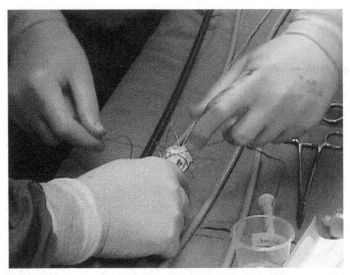

**Figure 17.3** A restraining silk suture is used to "back-load" the stent graft over the angiographic catheter.

and introducer were removed, and the introducer for the delivery sheath, with its tip trimmed, was used to pass the stent graft into deployment position.

The occluder was "back-loaded" into a trimmed sheath (i.e., loaded from the open end of the trimmed sheath toward the hub) that was 2F sizes smaller than the sheath used to deliver the graft segment. Because the proximal end of the occluder was oversewn, no guidewire or angiographic catheter was necessary. After the device was in the deployment position, renal angiography was performed before release. Because there were no restraining wires in this delivery system, exact positioning before deployment was mandatory. After deployment, the proximal bare stent and stent graft, in apposition with the aortic neck, were dilated with a 33-mm latex balloon (Boston Scientific Corp., Natick, MA) to the same diameter as the diameter of the adjacent arterial segment. Completion angiography was routinely performed. The procedure was completed with creation of a polytef femorofemoral bypass.

## Clinical results

Twenty-three patients underwent EVAR with custom aorto-uni-iliac Dacron grafts with internal stainless steel stents combined with contralateral common iliac artery occlusion and femorofemoral bypass. All patients were enrolled in a clinical trial that had institutional review board approval, and the devices were placed as part of an FDA-approved investigational device exemption (IDE G990024; A.G.H.).

**Table 17.1** Demographic and clinical data for 23 patients who received custom aorto-uni-iliac stent grafts in a US Food and Drug Administration-approved investigational device exemption protocol.

| Feature | Value* |
|---|---|
| Sex | |
|     Male | 22 (96%) |
|     Female | 1 (4%) |
| Age, years | 76 ± 1.3 (67–88) |
| AAA size, mm | 62.2 (44–75) |
| Ejection fraction, % | 43 ± 8 (14–63) |
| $FEV_1$ <1.0 L | 5 (22%) |
| CAD (irreversible ischemia) | 18 (78%) |
| Operative time, min | 186 ± 9.4 (80–370) |
| Length of stay, days | 3.2 ± 0.49 (2–11) |
| Follow-up interval, months | 19.6 ± 1.6 (14.3–37.5) |
| Wound infection | 1 (4.3%)[†] |

AAA, abdominal aortic aneurysm; CAD, coronary artery disease; $FEV_1$, forced expiratory volume in 1 s.
*Continuous data are presented as mean (range) or as mean ± SD (range); categorical data are presented as number of patients (% of patients).
[†]Infection occurred in one of 46 wounds (2.2%).

Patient demographic and clinical data are shown in Table 17.1: 96% of the patients were male; the mean size of the abdominal aortic aneurysm was 62.2 mm; for most patients, the comorbidity that was the highest surgical risk was either irreversible and uncorrectable coronary ischemia or pulmonary disease with a forced expiratory volume in 1 s of <1.0 L; length of hospital stay averaged 3.2 days; and follow-up averaged 19.6 months. All patients were followed up for a minimum of 14 months.

The anatomical characteristics for the 23 patients receiving custom devices are listed in Table 17.2. Proximal neck diameters up to 30 mm were treated with custom devices. Contralateral iliac artery occlusion was achieved with an occluder in 18 cases and with coil embolization or external iliac artery ligation in the remainder. Changes in the maximal transverse diameter of the aneurysm sac are shown in Table 17.3. Compared with the preoperative diameter, at 1 year after the procedure a significant decrease in mean (± SE) sac diameter was achieved: preoperative, 62.2 ± 1.56 mm ($n = 23$); at 1 year, 54.2 ± 2.54 mm ($n = 19$); $P < 0.01$. There were 10 endoleaks in 8 of 23 patients (35%) during the period of the study (Table 17.4). One patient had a recurrent type I endoleak (endoleaks 1 and 2 in Table 17.4), and a second patient had a type I endoleak, which was treated successfully, followed by a type II endoleak. Of the three type I endoleaks, one was successfully treated with a proximal extension, another sealed spontaneously, and the third was not treated. Of the six type II endoleaks, four sealed spontaneously, one was

**Table 17.2** Aortic, iliac artery, and stent graft dimensions and stent graft modifications in 23 patients who received custom aorto-uni-iliac stent grafts.

| Feature | Value* |
|---|---|
| Proximal aortic neck | |
| Diameter, mm | 24 (13–30) |
| Length, mm | 27 (10–65) |
| Distal diameter of common iliac artery, mm | 14 (10–18) |
| Stent graft | |
| Proximal diameter, mm | 28 (20–32) |
| Distal diameter, mm | 18 (10–24) |
| Length, mm | 149 (125–199) |
| Contralateral common iliac artery | |
| Diameter, mm | 15 (10–17) |
| Occluder diameter (18 patients), mm[†] | 19 (16–24) |
| Use of extension at initial operation | |
| Proximal | 6 (26.1%) |
| Distal | 7 (30.4%) |
| Proximal and distal | 1 (4.3%) |
| Bare stent for iliac artery dissection | 1 (4.3%) |

*Continuous data are presented as mean (range); categorical data as number of patients (% of patients).
[†]Three patients underwent coil embolization, and two underwent external iliac artery occlusion.

**Table 17.3** Maximal transverse diameter of abdominal aortic aneurysms at various intervals after treatment with custom aorto-uni-iliac stent grafts.

| Time, months | Patients, no. | Mean ± SE diameter, mm |
|---|---|---|
| 0 | 23 | 62.2 ± 1.56 |
| 1 | 21 | 61.0 ± 1.82 |
| 3 | 20 | 58.7 ± 2.30 |
| 6 | 19 | 58.5 ± 2.24 |
| 12 | 19 | 54.2 ± 2.54* |
| 18 | 11 | 52.7 ± 4.26* |
| 24 | 6 | 52.0 ± 8.44 |
| 25 | 3 | 44.0 ± 2.30 |
| 30 | 2 | 44.0 ± 5.65[†] |

*$P < 0.01$.
[†]$P < 0.03$.

treated successfully with transaortic coil embolization, and one was treated unsuccessfully with transaortic coil embolization and onyx glue injection. One type III endoleak, which occurred 28 months after the procedure, was successfully treated by placing a second aorto-uni-iliac device within the initial device.

**Table 17.4** Data on 10 endoleaks in 8 of 23 patients who received custom aorto-uni-iliac stent grafts.

| Endoleak no. | Date of operation, month/day/year | Initial AAA diameter, mm | Endoleak type | Diagnostic imaging | Treatment | Date of resolution, month/day/year | Latest follow-up | |
|---|---|---|---|---|---|---|---|---|
| | | | | | | | AAA diameter, mm | Postoperative month |
| 1 | 6/15/99 | 75 | Ia | Completion angiogram | None | 6/17/99 | 76 | 14 |
| 2 | 6/15/99 | 75 | Ia | CT scan | None | Not resolved | 92 | 14 |
| 3 | 7/13/99 | 60 | II | CT scan | Coil embolization | 7/6/01 | 55 | 37 |
| 4 | 6/27/00 | 72 | II | Completion angiogram | None | 7/24/00 | 60 | 24 |
| 5 | 8/23/00 | 56 | II | Completion angiogram | None | NA | 52 | 12 |
| 6 | 9/26/00 | 68 | II | Completion angiogram | None | 10/30/00 | 59 | 23 |
| 7 | 9/26/00 | 68 | I | CT scan | Proximal extension | 9/27/01 | 59 | 23 |
| 8 | 10/11/00 | 74 | II | CT scan | Coil embolization; glue injection | Not resolved | 76 | 20 |
| 9 | 3/5/01 | 67 | II | Completion angiogram | None | Not resolved | 60 | 14 |
| 10 | 7/21/00 | 54 | III | CT scan | Second graft within initial graft | 11/24/02 | 39 | 30 |

AAA, abdominal aortic aneurysm; CT, computed tomographic; NA, not available.

**Table 17.5** Secondary procedures in 5 of 23 patients who received custom aorto-uni-iliac stent grafts.

| Procedure | Interventions, no. |
|---|---|
| Conversion to open repair | 0 |
| Proximal extension for migration without endoleak | 1 |
| Proximal extension for type I endoleak | 1 |
| Embolization/glue for type II endoleak | 3* |
| Second graft within initial graft for type III endoleak | 1 |

*Three interventions in two patients: both were treated with coil embolization; one was also treated with onyx glue injection.

**Table 17.6** Cause of death, 1999–2002, for 9 of 23 patients (39%) who received custom aorto-uni-iliac stent grafts.

| Death no. | Age, years | Date of operation, month/day/year | Date of death, month/day/year | Follow-up interval, month | AAA diameter, mm Initial | Latest | Cause of death |
|---|---|---|---|---|---|---|---|
| 1 | 75 | 6/15/99 | 5/19/02 | 35 | 75 | 92* | CHF |
| 2 | 76 | 7/28/99 | 7/28/99 | 0 | 63 | 63 | Respiratory arrest |
| 3 | 72 | 9/08/99 | 5/01/01 | 21 | 55 | 47 | COPD |
| 4 | 76 | 10/19/99 | 11/01/00 | 13 | 59 | 58 | CAD |
| 5 | 72 | 2/10/00 | 7/27/00 | 6 | 44 | 38 | MSOF |
| 6 | 82 | 3/29/00 | 8/1/00 | 6 | 64 | 63 | CHF |
| 7 | 69 | 8/17/00 | 4/7/02 | 20 | 65 | 60 | Cirrhosis |
| 8 | 69 | 3/20/01 | 10/15/02 | 20 | 67 | 60 | COPD |
| 9 | 70 | 7/21/99 | 12/29/02 | 41 | 56 | 40 | Lung cancer |

AAA, abdominal aortic aneurysm; CAD, coronary artery disease; CHF, congestive heart failure; COPD, chronic obstructive pulmonary disease; MSOF, multisystem organ failure.
*Patient had type I endoleak.

Secondary procedures in the 23 patients during the study are summarized in Table 17.5. In addition to the interventions for endoleaks, one patient underwent placement of a proximal extension for distal device migration without endoleak. Of the 23 patients who had primary procedures, 5 patients (22%) required 6 secondary interventions. No patient required conversion to open repair. The causes of death for 9 of the 23 patients (39%) during the 3-year study period are listed in Table 17.6. No deaths were related to aneurysmal rupture or to conversion to open surgical repair. The chronology of death is summarized in Table 17.7.

**Table 17.7** Distribution of 9 deaths among 23 patients who received custom aorto-uni-iliac stent grafts.

| Time of death | Deaths | |
|---|---|---|
| | No. of patients | % of patients |
| Perioperative | 1 | 4.3 |
| Year postoperative | | |
| 1 | 2 | 8.7 |
| 2 | 5 | 21.7 |
| 3 | 1 | 4.3 |
| Total | 9 | 39.0 |

## Summary

Twenty-three high-risk surgical patients underwent EVAR with custom aorto-uni-iliac devices. All procedures successfully excluded the aneurysm. Secondary procedures for endoleak or stent graft migration, however, were required in 22% of the patients. In the majority of patients who died, the same comorbidity responsible for the high surgical risk was also responsible for death.

## References

1 Dotter CT. Transluminally-placed coilspring endarterial tube grafts: long-term patency in canine popliteal artery. *Invest Radiol* 1969; **4**: 329–32.

2 Volodos NL, Karpovich IP, Troyan VI *et al*. Endovascular stented grafts for thoracic, abdominal aortic, and iliac arterial disease: clinical experience in the Ukraine from 1985. *Semin Intervent Radiol* 1998; **15**: 89–95.

3 Parodi JC, Palmaz JC, Barone HD. Transfemoral intraluminal graft implantation for abdominal aortic aneurysms. *Ann Vasc Surg* 1991; **5**: 491–9.

4 Ivancev K, Resch T, Brunkwall J *et al*. Endoluminal repair of abdominal aortic aneurysms: a critical reappraisal after a three-and-a-half year experience. *Semin Intervent Radiol* 1998; **15**: 97–108.

5 Chuter TA, Reilly LM, Faruqi RM *et al*. Endovascular aneurysm repair in high-risk patients. *J Vasc Surg* 2000; **31**: 122–33.

6 Yusuf SW, Whitaker SC, Chuter TA *et al*. Early results of endovascular aortic aneurysm surgery with aortouniiliac graft, contralateral iliac occlusion, and femorofemoral bypass. *J Vasc Surg* 1997; **25**: 165–72.

7 Gordon MK, Lawrence-Brown MM, Hartley D *et al*. A self-expanding endoluminal graft for treatment of aneurysms: results through the development phase. *Aust N Z J Surg* 1996; **66**: 621–5.

8 Resch T, Ivancev K, Brunkwall J *et al*. Distal migration of stent-grafts after endovascular repair of abdominal aortic aneurysms. *J Vasc Interv Radiol* 1999; **10**: 257–64.

9 Malina M, Brunkwall J, Lindblad B, Resch T, Ivancev K. Endovascular management of the juxtarenal aortic aneurysm: can uncovered stents safely cross the renal arteries? *Semin Vasc Surg* 1999; **12**: 182–91.

10 Lawrence-Brown M, Sieunarine K, Hartley D, Van Schie G, Anderson J. Should an anchor stent cross the renal artery orifices when placing an endoluminal graft for abdominal aortic aneurysms? In: Greenhalgh RM, ed. *Indications in Vascular and Endovascular Surgery*. London: WB Saunders, 1998: 261–9.

# PART IV

---

# Intraoperative ancillary procedures

# CHAPTER 18

# Use of intravascular ultrasonography in endovascular intervention

Jonathan D. Woody, MD, George E. Kopchok, BS,
James T. Lee, MD, Rodney A. White, MD

## Introduction

Numerous excellent vascular imaging techniques are readily available, including angiography, computed tomographic angiography, magnetic resonance angiography, angioscopy, and intravascular ultrasonography (IVUS). Each technique provides unique vascular anatomical information and each has its own indications, advantages, and disadvantages. All the techniques have been continually improved and they complement each other well, but IVUS has evolved into an essential component of vascular imaging and is especially important in endovascular therapy. Although IVUS requires additional equipment and personnel, it is an invaluable adjunct to conventional imaging because it provides sensitive, real-time imaging for endovascular intervention and simultaneously decreases exposure to contrast agents and radiation. Even though the initial cost of the catheters may be a deterrent to their use, the cost of an additional endoluminal graft component or a secondary intervention that may be prevented by the use of IVUS far outweighs the costs associated with the use of IVUS.

## Intravascular ultrasonographic design and function

In the 1950s, IVUS was first used to image cardiac chamber size and motion [1,2]. A rotating ultrasound beam was developed in the 1970s that allowed for the acquisition of intraluminal, 360° cross-sectional images [3–6]. The plane of imaging is perpendicular to the long axis of the catheter and provides a full 360° image of the blood vessel. Currently, intravascular ultrasonographic catheters are manufactured by several companies and are available in various frequencies. Smaller diameter catheters use higher frequency transducers and provide greater image resolution but sacrifice depth of beam penetration. Conversely, larger diameter catheters use lower frequency transducers and provide greater depth of beam penetration but sacrifice image resolution. Typically, 30-MHz catheters are used for coronary arteries and 12.5- or 20-MHz catheters are used for peripheral vessels.

Modern intravascular ultrasonographic catheters come in two configurations, the rotating mirror catheter and the multiple array transducer. The rotating mirror catheter consists of a rotating mirror and, in the tip of the catheter, a transducer that is rotated by a cable that runs inside the catheter. This type of catheter is attached to a motor drive unit that transmits the image to the ultrasonographic monitor. Before this catheter is used, saline is injected into the imaging chamber. The Sonicath catheter (Boston Scientific Corp., Natick, MA) is an example of a rotating mirror catheter. The multiple array transducer has an integrated circuit in the tip of the catheter and does not require any preparation because there is no imaging chamber in the catheter. The Visions catheter (Volcano Therapeutics, Inc., Rancho Cordova, CA) is an example of a multiple array transducer catheter.

Intravascular ultrasonographic catheters are inserted through a sheath that can be placed into a vessel by means of open surgical exposure or percutaneous puncture. These catheters should be inserted over a guidewire, which provides better control of the catheter and allows for smooth passage of the catheter through tortuous or stenotic vessels. The catheters can be passed over guidewires ranging in size from 0.009 to 0.038 inches.

## Clinical applications of intravascular ultrasonography

IVUS can delineate many vascular anatomical characteristics, including the following: lumen diameter; cross-sectional area; wall thickness; lesion length, shape, and volume; lesion position within the lumen (concentric or eccentric); lesion type (fibrous or calcific); presence and extent of flap, dissection, or ulceration; and presence and volume of thrombus. Information from IVUS about a particular location within a blood vessel can be critical in planning or evaluating an endovascular intervention. For critical assessment of endovascular intervention, more information is required than can be provided by the luminal silhouette obtained with angiography.

### Percutaneous transluminal angioplasty and stenting

IVUS is a useful tool when used with percutaneous transluminal angioplasty. Before the intervention, IVUS is used to distinguish between calcified and fibrous lesions and between concentric and eccentric lesions. These features are believed to be important predictors of postintervention complications and late failures [7].

After percutaneous transluminal angioplasty, IVUS can document dissection (Figure 18.1) and plaque fracture, which may necessitate stent placement. Incomplete stent expansion, which may lead to early complications such as stent thrombosis and migration, can be missed with angiography in up to 40% of cases [8]. Likewise, overexpansion may lead to vessel wall injury and subsequent rupture or to the development of intimal hyperplasia and restenosis [9]. With IVUS, incomplete stent expansion is apparent as a gap between the stent and the arterial wall, thus alerting the interventionalist to the need for

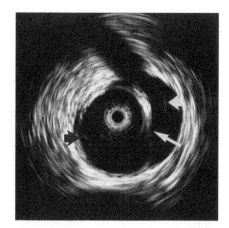

**Figure 18.1** Intravascular ultrasonographic image shows aortic dissection. The false lumen (short white arrow) supplies the celiac artery. Long white arrow, septum; black arrow, true lumen.

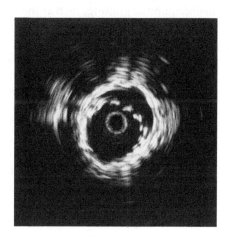

**Figure 18.2** Intravascular ultrasonographic image shows incomplete expansion of a stent graft in the iliac artery.

further balloon dilation of the stent (Figure 18.2). IVUS also allows for precise and accurate sizing of the vessel so that the appropriate stent and balloon size may be chosen. Several authors have demonstrated that balloon size is frequently underestimated by angiography alone and that IVUS predicts optimal balloon size more accurately than angiography [10,11]. Further, IVUS effectively documents the adequacy of the primary intervention and establishes the need for any additional intervention [12–14].

## Endoluminal grafting

With the explosion of interest in endoluminal stent graft techniques for the treatment of aneurysmal disease, IVUS has again proved to be invaluable. When compared with angiography and computed tomography, IVUS is the most accurate method of determining the aneurysm neck size and the device fixation site [15]. At Harbor-UCLA Medical Center (Torrence, CA), spiral computed tomography is the predominant method of preoperative imaging for endoluminal aneurysm cases, and it has been accurate in selecting appropriate candidates for endoluminal grafting and in planning device size and selection before intervention. In most cases, preoperative angiography is no longer performed. Still, discrepancies between preoperative sizing on spiral computed tomography and the intraoperative assessment with IVUS necessitate at least some change in plan for up to 20% of endoluminal graft patients [16]. In these cases, without the aid of IVUS, undersized devices would have been deployed that may have led to poor outcomes. Given the anatomical complexities of aneurysmal disease and the importance of accurate graft sizing and placement, this is not surprising. We believe that in the early phase of endoluminal graft development, the more information available to the interventionalist, the higher the likelihood of a successful outcome for the patient.

The real-time imaging of IVUS easily locates landmarks that are important in endoluminal grafting, such as the mesenteric and renal vessels (Figures 18.3 and 18.4) in abdominal aortic aneurysm cases and the aortic arch vessels in thoracic aortic aneurysm cases. In addition, the "pull-back" method of imaging allows for the accurate measurement of luminal length, which further enhances the ability to properly select and place endoluminal grafts. ("Pull-back" length is measured by withdrawing the catheter from the proximal to the distal points of interest, thereby determining the length of stent or stent graft to cover the desired segment of vessel.) IVUS also decreases the amount of contrast medium and radiation to which the patient and staff are exposed. In several patients with marginal renal function, IVUS has enabled us to implant endoluminal grafts without the use of any contrast medium. In more complicated cases, such as in patients with large or tortuous iliac vessels, IVUS enables accurate, real-time evaluation of potential fixation points

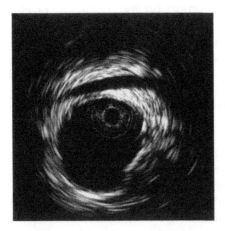

**Figure 18.3** Intravascular ultrasonographic image shows the left renal vein crossing anterior to the aorta.

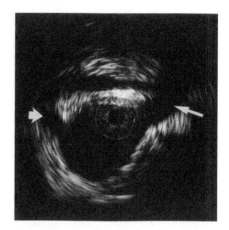

**Figure 18.4** Intravascular ultrasonographic image shows the left renal vein crossing anterior to the aorta and the orifices of the right (short arrow) and left (long arrow) renal arteries.

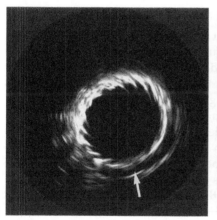

a

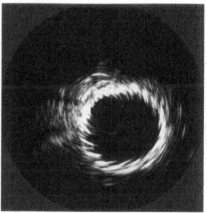

b

**Figure 18.5** Intravascular ultrasonographic images. (a) Gap (arrow) between the stent graft and aortic wall. (b) Good apposition between the stent graft and the aortic wall after balloon dilatation.

proximal to the hypogastric artery. In many cases, this may eliminate the need for coil embolization or occlusion of the hypogastric artery.

As with angioplasty and stent deployment, IVUS allows for clear visualization of device fixation sites and confirmation of whether an appropriate seal has been obtained. If the arterial wall pulsates independently of the stent graft, further balloon dilation of the graft is needed to ensure adequate device fixation and to prevent an endoleak from occurring at the attachment site (Figure 18.5). IVUS is also useful when the exact location of the renal artery orifice is in question. IVUS allows for the precise localization of aortic branch vessels, whereas aortography is sometimes less than optimal for precise localization of these vessels.

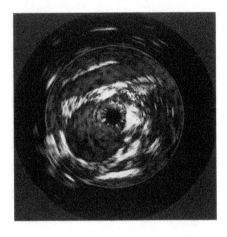

**Figure 18.6** Intravascular ultrasonography with color flow imaging shows flow in the left renal vein anterior to the aorta and in the left renal artery.

## Future perspective

Endovascular therapeutics continue to evolve and improve in technique and application. IVUS is an important adjunct to other imaging methods and is becoming increasingly useful in endovascular aneurysm repair. Further refinement of catheter technology is leading to the development of catheters with smaller diameters. Another intriguing area of research is the development of color flow technology for intravascular ultrasonographic catheters. Color flow capabilities allow for the delineation of the vessel lumen in cases in which this is difficult to accomplish with conventional gray-scale technology (Figure 18.6). Perhaps more importantly, color flow imaging may be useful for locating defects in the walls of endoluminal grafts and for assessing all types of endoleaks and guiding their treatment. Although many centers have limited or no experience with IVUS, its use is becoming broader because of the increasing need for accurate assessment of vessel dimensions and characteristics to ensure appropriate sizing and fixation of endoluminal grafts.

## Conclusion

IVUS is easy to use and it provides valuable information. As endovascular techniques evolve, IVUS will be increasingly important in endovascular imaging. New developments, especially color flow imaging with IVUS, will provide a greater degree of accuracy and utility in endovascular imaging and will allow IVUS to become an increasingly significant adjunct in endovascular intervention.

## References

1  Bom N, ten Hoff H, Lancee CT, Gussenhoven WJ, Bosch JG. Early and recent intraluminal ultrasound devices. *Int J Card Imaging* 1989; **4**: 79–88.

2 Cieszynski T. Intracardiac method for the investigation of structure of the heart with the aid of ultrasonics. *Arch Immun Ther Exp (Warsz)* 1960; **8**: 551–7 [in Polish].

3 Kossof G. Diagnostic applications of ultrasound in cardiology. *Australas Radiol* 1966; **10**: 101–6.

4 Carleton RA, Sessions RW, Graettinger JS. Diameter of heart measured by intracavitary ultrasound. *Med Res Eng* 1969; **8**: 28–32

5 Frazin L, Talano JV, Stephanides L *et al.* Esophageal echocardiography. *Circulation* 1976; **54**: 102–8.

6 Bom N, Lancee CT, Van Egmond FC. An ultrasonic intracardiac scanner. *Ultrasonics* 1972; **10**: 72–6.

7 The SH, Gussenhoven EJ, Zhong Y *et al.* Effect of balloon angioplasty on femoral artery evaluated with intravascular ultrasound imaging. *Circulation* 1992; **86**: 483–93.

8 Buckley CJ, Arko FR, Lee S *et al.* Intravascular ultrasound scanning improves long-term patency of iliac lesions treated with balloon angioplasty and primary stenting. *J Vasc Surg* 2002; **35**: 316–23.

9 Busquet J. The current role of vascular stents. *Int Angiol* 1993; **12**: 206–13.

10 Roubin GS, Douglas JS Jr, King SB III *et al.* Influence of balloon size on initial success, acute complications, and restenosis after percutaneous transluminal coronary angioplasty: a prospective randomized study. *Circulation* 1988; **78**: 557–65.

11 Nichols AB, Smith R, Berke AD, Shlofmitz RA, Powers ER. Importance of balloon size in coronary angioplasty. *J Am Coll Cardiol* 1989; **13**: 1094–100.

12 Scoccianti M, Verbin CS, Kopchok GE *et al.* Intravascular ultrasound guidance for peripheral vascular interventions. *J Endovasc Surg* 1994; **1**: 71–80.

13 Diethrich EB. Endovascular treatment of abdominal aortic occlusive disease: the impact of stents and intravascular ultrasound imaging. *Eur J Vasc Surg* 1993; **7**: 228–36.

14 Cavaye DM, Diethrich EB, Santiago OJ *et al.* Intravascular ultrasound imaging: an essential component of angioplasty assessment and vascular stent deployment. *Int Angiol* 1993; **12**: 214–20.

15 White RA, Scoccianti M, Back M, Kopchok G, Donayre C. Innovations in vascular imaging: arteriography, three-dimensional CT scans, and two- and three-dimensional intravascular ultrasound evaluation of an abdominal aortic aneurysm. *Ann Vasc Surg* 1994; **8**: 285–9.

16 Nishanian G, Kopchok GE, Donayre CE, White RA. The impact of intravascular ultrasound (IVUS) on endovascular interventions. *Semin Vasc Surg* 1999; **12**: 285–99.

# CHAPTER 19

# Intentional occlusion of the internal iliac artery to facilitate endovascular repair of aortoiliac aneurysms

**Alfio Carroccio, MD, Peter L. Faries, MD, Michael L. Marin, MD, Osvaldo Juniti Yano, MD, Larry H. Hollier, MD**

## Introduction

Aortic aneurysms often extend beyond the aortic bifurcation and involve the iliac arteries. Modification of the endovascular approach for this disease process often necessitates deployment of the endograft near the common iliac artery bifurcation. Endovascular treatment of aortoiliac aneurysms and subsequent endovascular modifications involve certain considerations. One such consideration is the deliberate or unplanned interruption of the internal iliac arteries, which, along with its potential consequences, is described in this chapter.

## Background

Interruption of the internal iliac arteries is not a new technique. For years, ligation or embolization has been used for the management of post-traumatic hemorrhage [1], obstetric hemorrhage [2,3], and intraoperative hemorrhage. Most reports have focused on the success of this approach and discussed the potential consequences, but studies investigating the outcome in long-term follow-up have been limited. In addition, a majority of the populations reported were young, so that the possible added risk of atherosclerotic disease was not significant.

In 1987, Iliopoulos *et al.* [4] reported on 11 patients with ischemic complications after aortoiliac reconstruction or spontaneous aortoiliac thrombosis. Bilateral acute ischemia of the internal iliac arteries resulted in paralysis, buttock necrosis, anal and bladder sphincteric dysfunction, or colorectal ischemia. The mortality rate was 100% when buttock necrosis developed. These complications occurred despite patent bypass grafts to the iliac or femoral vessels, suggesting that it is essential to maintain patency of the internal iliac vessels in all aortoiliac reconstructions.

Later Iliopoulos *et al.* [5] designed a study to assess the major sources of collateral supply to the internal iliac arterial bed. Peak systolic internal iliac artery and radial artery pressures were measured before and after clamping a patent internal iliac artery and after additional clamping of the contralateral internal iliac artery, the contralateral external iliac artery, or the ipsilateral external iliac artery, selectively and in combinations. These procedures were performed in 10 patients who had aortoiliac aneurysm or occlusive disease. The data suggest that branches of the ipsilateral external iliac artery–femoral artery system provide a better collateral pathway than the contralateral internal iliac artery. They also suggest that it is important to relieve occlusive disease in the ipsilateral external iliac artery–femoral artery system if a patent internal iliac artery is ligated or bypassed during aortoiliac reconstructions. Conversely, it is especially important to preserve perfusion in a patent internal iliac artery in a patient with compromised ipsilateral external iliac artery–femoral artery runoff.

## Interruption of the iliac artery

The extent of an infrarenal aortic aneurysm is quite variable. Although the aneurysm may be limited to the aortic segment, extension to the iliac arteries is common. Therefore, a consideration for the endovascular management of aneurysmal disease in the aortoiliac segment must be the anatomical variation among patients. The presence of iliac aneurysm, ectasia, or tortuosity makes selection of the appropriate device critical. In these situations, the distal end of the endograft must be positioned within the iliac artery at a location where the fixation of the graft can completely exclude the aneurysm sac (Figure 19.1).

Two types of stent grafts extend into the iliac arteries. When a bifurcated stent graft is used, a limb from the aortic segment is anchored in each iliac artery (Figure 19.2). When an aorto-uni-iliac stent graft is used, the contralateral common iliac artery is occluded and an extra-anatomic femorofemoral bypass is constructed to perfuse the contralateral pelvis and limb (Figure 19.3).

Sacrifice of one or both of the internal iliac arteries is required in situations in the following list.

1 The extent of the common iliac artery aneurysm on a particular side results in an inadequate length of acceptable vessel proximal to the internal iliac artery takeoff to completely seal the distal portion of the graft.

2 There is aneurysmal dilatation of the internal iliac artery.

3 The common iliac artery is severely tortuous, calcified, or narrowed, so that there is a high likelihood of complication in delivery and positioning of the graft; consequently, the preferred procedure may include contralateral extension of the graft to the external iliac artery and subsequent femorofemoral bypass.

4 Emergent repair is required, with no time for creating an individualized device, including a unifemoral extension.

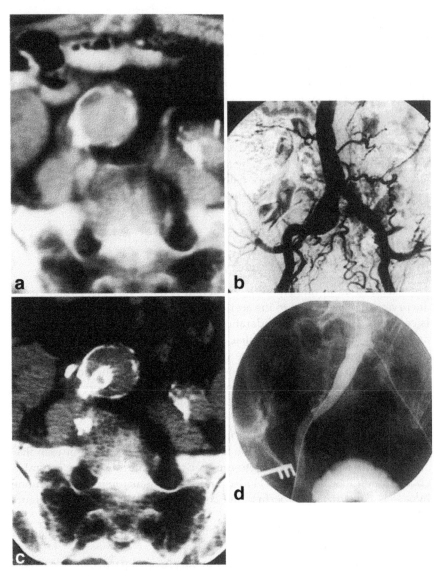

**Figure 19.1** Iliac artery aneurysm. Preoperative computed tomographic (CT) scan (a) and angiogram (b) show aneurysm of the common iliac artery proximal to the takeoff of the internal iliac artery. Postoperative CT scan (c) and angiogram (d) show the excluded aneurysm.

Alone or in combination, these four situations require sacrifice of one or both of the internal iliac arteries for endovascular therapy of aortoiliac aneurysmal disease. The risks and consequences of such sacrifice must prove worthwhile before this concept becomes more accepted.

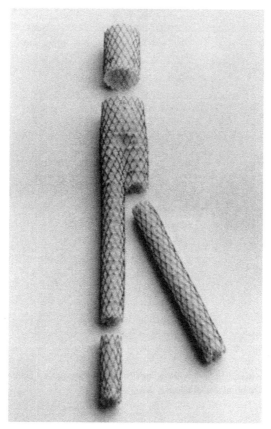

**Figure 19.2** Multimodular bifurcated stent graft (AneuRx; Medtronic, Inc., Minneapolis, MN).

## Predictive factors for pelvic ischemia

To demonstrate whether there were any predictive factors for clinical pelvic ischemia, we compared clinical outcome with angiographic findings in patients who had undergone unilateral or bilateral intentional occlusion of the internal iliac arteries to facilitate endovascular repair of their aortoiliac aneurysms. During a 6-year follow-up, the clinical sequelae in 103 patients were recorded (unpubl. data). To allow time for pelvic collateralization, the intentional occlusions of the internal iliac artery were performed at least 3 weeks before definitive repair of the endovascular aneurysm. Occlusion of the internal iliac artery was achieved in 100% of the patients by either selective catheter-directed coil embolization or direct coverage of the vessel orifice by an endovascular graft. None of the patients in this study had angiographic evidence of significant visceral arterial occlusive disease before the procedure. To facilitate data interpretation and to objectively correlate the preoperative

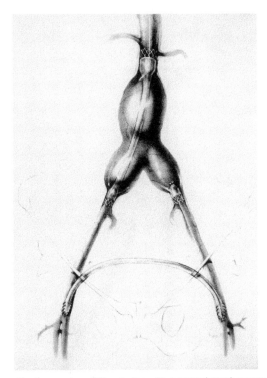

**Figure 19.3** Schematic of an aorto-uni-iliac device with a contralateral common iliac occluder and extra-anatomic femorofemoral bypass.

angiograms with the clinical presentation of pelvic ischemia, the following classification was developed: class 0, no symptoms; class I, nonlimiting claudication with exercise; class II, new-onset impotence with moderate to severe buttock pain, leading to physical limitations with exercise; and class III, buttock rest pain or colonic ischemia (or both).

One investigator performed a blinded assessment of collateral branches (Figure 19.4) to and from the internal iliac arteries on preoperative and intra-operative angiograms. The specific arterial branches studied were the following:

1 the fourth and fifth lumbar branches to the iliolumbar artery
2 the inferior mesenteric artery to the superior hemorrhoidal artery
3 the superior hemorrhoidal artery to the middle hemorrhoidal artery
4 the middle sacral branches to the lateral sacral branches
5 the superior gluteal artery to the lateral circumflex femoral artery
6 the deep and superficial circumflex iliac arteries to the external iliac artery
7 the obturator artery to the inferior epigastric artery
8 the internal pudendal artery to the inferior rectal artery, which sometimes anastomoses with the deep femoral artery (medial circumflex femoral artery)

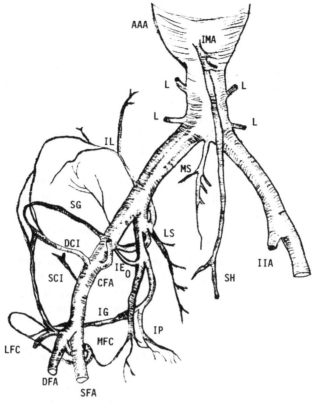

**Figure 19.4** Illustration of pertinent pelvic circulation. AAA, abdominal aortic aneurysm; CFA, common femoral artery; DCI, deep circumflex iliac artery; DFA, deep femoral artery; IE, inferior epigastric artery; IG, inferior gluteal artery; IIA, internal iliac artery; IL, iliolumbar artery; IMA, inferior mesenteric artery; IP, inferior pudendal artery; LFC, lateral femoral circumflex artery; L, lumbar artery; LS, lateral sacral artery; MFC, medial femoral circumflex artery; MS, middle sacral artery; O, obturator artery; SFA, superficial femoral artery; SH, superior hemorrhoidal artery; SCI, superior circumflex iliac artery; SG, superior gluteal artery. (Reprinted from Yano OJ, Morrissey N, Eisen L *et al.*, Intentional internal iliac artery occlusion to facilitate endovascular repair of aortoiliac aneurysms, *J Vasc Surg* 2001; **34**: 204–11, Copyright 2001, with permission from the Society for Vascular Surgery and the American Association for Vascular Surgery.)

9 the central anatomical system, which corresponds to the numerous collaterals between the superior, middle, and inferior sacral branches (middle rectal, inferior vesicle, ovarian, and uterine arteries)

To simplify the interpretation of the rich pelvic vascular network, the pelvic circulation was classified as contralateral or ipsilateral in relation to the internal iliac artery planned for occlusion. In addition, the appearance of the pelvic vessels, including the caliber of the artery and whether a particular collateral crossed the pelvic midline, was recorded for each patient.

Of the 103 patients in this study, 22 (21%) presented with some symptoms of pelvic ischemia (16 unilateral; 6 bilateral). Five patients with class I ischemia improved and became asymptomatic within 1 year, and one patient's classification was changed from class II to class I when symptoms improved. Seventeen patients (16%) had chronic pelvic claudication. Interestingly, there were two findings identified on the preoperative or intraoperative angiograms of the 17 patients who had chronic pelvic claudication: (1) evidence of chronic pelvic ischemia manifested by stenosis of the contralateral internal iliac artery origin (≥70% of the patients), nonopacification of at least three named branches of the internal iliac artery, and the presence of newly developed collaterals (63% of the patients), and (2) small-caliber, diseased, or absent medial and lateral circumflex femoral arteries (ascending deep femoral branches) ipsilateral to the side of the internal iliac artery occlusion (25% of the patients).

One patient with class III ischemia died of cardiovascular collapse associated with colon ischemia. This patient's preoperative angiogram showed a normal superior mesenteric artery and celiac trunk, an occluded inferior mesenteric artery at its origin, and a large Riolan arcade, which was patent to the left colon. The superior mesenteric and celiac arteries should be confirmed as being anatomically normal before unilateral or bilateral occlusion of the internal iliac artery.

Although the study has limitations both in population size, given the potential collateral variability, and in the need for a better protocol for pelvic arterial evaluation, the data illustrate the importance of an adequate assessment of the individual collateral arterial supply to the pelvis. The findings also suggest that, despite the complexity of the pelvic arterial circulation, careful preoperative evaluation of the visceral, pelvic, and upper thigh circulation should be performed so that chronic pelvic ischemia can be anticipated and perhaps avoided before occlusion of the internal iliac artery. Although the majority of patients have adequate collateral pelvic vessels that can compensate for the sacrifice of one internal iliac artery, it is not prudent to assume the safety of random occlusion of the internal iliac artery in patients with aneurysmal disease.

## Outcomes after occlusion of the internal iliac artery

Supporters of internal iliac artery occlusion include Wolpert *et al.* [6] who retrospectively reviewed patients who had internal iliac artery embolization for endovascular repair of abdominal aortic aneurysms. Patients underwent unilateral or staged bilateral coil embolizations with an approximate 1-week interval between procedures. Follow-up ranged from 1 to 12 months. Of the 65 patients who underwent endovascular abdominal aortic aneurysm (AAA) repair, 18 patients (28%) required internal iliac artery embolization. Seven of these patients (39%) underwent bilateral embolization. There were no episodes of clinically evident bowel ischemia. Hip or buttock claudication had occurred in approximately 50% of patients with persistent but improved symptoms at 6 months. Only two patients noted worsening of erectile function postoperatively.

Similarly, Criado *et al.* [7] retrospectively reviewed 156 patients who underwent stent graft repair of abdominal aortic aneurysms. Coil embolization of one or both internal iliac arteries was undertaken when the diameter of the common iliac artery was >20 mm, which enabled limb endograft extension to the external iliac artery. Thirty-nine of 156 patients (25%) were selected for coil embolization of one ($n = 28$) or both ($n = 11$) internal iliac arteries. The interventions were performed before ($n = 31$) or during ($n = 8$) the stent graft procedure. One patient had erectile dysfunction, and five patients (13%) had buttock claudication after unilateral occlusion. Serious ischemic complications were not observed.

Karch *et al.* [8] reported an intentional occlusion in 16% of their 96 patients. Two patients underwent intentional occlusion of one internal iliac artery and subsequent unintentional occlusion of the contralateral internal iliac artery because of a traumatic iliac dissection. Both had postoperative abdominal pain and distention; rectosigmoid ischemia was evident through colonoscopy. Conservative treatment with bowel rest and broad-spectrum antibiotics was successful despite the nonstaged bilateral occlusion.

Lee *et al.* [9] studied the long-term functional outcome after unilateral internal iliac artery occlusion during elective endovascular stent graft repair of aortoiliac aneurysms. Of the 157 consecutive patients, 23 (15%) had unilateral internal iliac artery occlusion and none had bilateral occlusions. Among the 23 patients, two groups were identified: 10 patients (43%) had planned and 13 patients (57%) had unplanned or inadvertent occlusions. Nine of the 23 patients (39%), five with planned occlusions and four with unplanned occlusions, reported significant symptoms of hip and buttock claudication ipsilateral to their occluded internal iliac arteries. The symptoms were universally noted on postoperative day 1. Although eight of the nine patients (89%) improved, one (11%) did not. Among those whose symptoms improved, the mean time to improvement was 15 weeks, but a plateau thereafter resulted in a net decrement from baseline. The authors concluded that, although most patients with symptoms had some improvement, none returned to their baseline level of activity. Despite this, when questioned whether in retrospect they would undergo the procedure again, all patients indicated that they would still choose endovascular repair over conventional open repair.

Mehta *et al.* [10] reported on a population of 154 patients with abdominal aortic aneurysms ($n = 66$), iliac aneurysms ($n = 28$), or aortoiliac aneurysms ($n = 60$) that required interruption of one ($n = 134$) or both ($n = 20$) internal iliac arteries as part of their endovascular ($n = 107$) or open ($n = 47$) repair. There were no cases of buttock necrosis, ischemic colitis requiring laparotomy, or death when one or both internal iliac arteries were interrupted. The authors believed that other comorbid factors, such as shock, distal embolization, or the failure to preserve collateral branches from the external iliac and femoral arteries, may have contributed to the morbidity in other reports of internal iliac artery interruption.

In the preceding studies, depending on the device, approach, and aggressiveness of the authors, the intentional occlusion of the internal iliac arteries was necessary in 6–28% of the endovascular repairs. Unilateral occlusion was intended in 6–18% of the endograft repairs; at institutions that used bilateral, intentional, staged interruption of the internal iliac arteries, the procedure was performed in 7–11% of the repairs. In all the studies, the most common complication was buttock claudication, which occurred in 13–50% of the cases, with improvement in the long term. Erectile dysfunction occurred less frequently, in 2.5–5% of the cases.

## Summary

Despite our aggressive approach to complex aortoiliac aneurysms, careful preoperative imaging tests are recommended for assessing all possible sources of collateral vessels that can be recruited to provide perfusion to the pelvis from visceral, pelvic, and upper thigh circulations after the occlusion of one or both of the internal iliac arteries. Because atherosclerosis in the pelvic circulation seems to impede the development of new collaterals and promote the underdevelopment of the ipsilateral femoral circulation, we recommend that extreme caution and good clinical judgment should be exercised before intentional occlusion of one or both of the internal iliac arteries.

## References

1 van Urk H, Perlberger RR, Muller H. Selective arterial embolization for control of traumatic pelvic hemorrhage. *Surgery* 1978; **83**: 133–7.

2 Evans S, McShane P. The efficacy of internal iliac artery ligation in obstetric hemorrhage. *Surg Gynecol Obstet* 1985; **160**: 250–3.

3 Hansch E, Chitkara U, McAlpine J, El-Sayed Y, Dake MD, Razavi MK. Pelvic arterial embolization for control of obstetric hemorrhage: a five-year experience. *Am J Obstet Gynecol* 1999; **180**: 1454–60.

4 Iliopoulos JI, Howanitz PE, Pierce GE, Kueshkerian SM, Thomas JH, Hermreck AS. The critical hypogastric circulation. *Am J Surg* 1987; **154**: 671–5.

5 Iliopoulos JI, Hermreck AS, Thomas JH, Pierce GE. Hemodynamics of the hypogastric arterial circulation. *J Vasc Surg* 1989; **9**: 637–41.

6 Wolpert LM, Dittrich KP, Hallisey MJ et al. Hypogastric artery embolization in endovascular abdominal aortic aneurysm repair. *J Vasc Surg* 2001; **33**: 1193–8.

7 Criado FJ, Wilson EP, Velazquez OC et al. Safety of coil embolization of the internal iliac artery in endovascular grafting of abdominal aortic aneurysms. *J Vasc Surg* 2000; **32**: 684–8.

8 Karch LA, Hodgson KJ, Mattos MA, Bohannon WT, Ramsay DE, McLafferty RB. Adverse consequences of internal iliac artery occlusion during endovascular repair of abdominal aortic aneurysms. *J Vasc Surg* 2000; **32**: 676–83.

9  Lee WA, O'Dorisio J, Wolf YG, Hill BB, Fogarty TJ, Zarins CK. Outcome after unilateral hypogastric artery occlusion during endovascular aneurysm repair. *J Vasc Surg* 2001; **33**: 921–6.

10  Mehta M, Veith FJ, Ohki T *et al*. Unilateral and bilateral hypogastric artery interruption during aortoiliac aneurysm repair in 154 patients: a relatively innocuous procedure. *J Vasc Surg* 2001; **33**(Suppl): S27–32.

# CHAPTER 20

# Arterial access for endovascular aneurysm repair

**Timothy A.M. Chuter, MD**

## Introduction

In the early days of endovascular aneurysm repair, the topic of arterial access was very important because the repair systems were too large to traverse small iliac arteries and too blunt or inflexible to traverse tortuous iliac arteries. In those days, the commonest cause of failed endovascular aneurysm repair was failure to reach the aorta from a femoral insertion site, and one of the commonest complications was iliac artery rupture [1].

Various maneuvers were developed to overcome these limitations [2]. Some of these tricks will always be useful for anatomical challenges, but rapid advances in delivery system design are making most of the maneuvers unnecessary. Tapered, trackable delivery systems now follow stiff guidewires through tortuous iliac arteries, and 18F and 20F delivery systems are generally small enough and smooth enough to be pushed through all but diffusely stenotic external iliac arteries. Large-caliber delivery systems, such as those of the Talent (Medtronic, Inc., Minneapolis, MN) and AneuRx (Medtronic, Inc.) devices, and delivery systems of thoracic aortic stent grafts, however, still require adjunctive maneuvers of this kind.

## Iliac artery tortuosity

In most cases, the iliac arteries can be straightened using a stiff guidewire and a trackable delivery system (Figure 20.1). They may look unusual when skewered on a very stiff guidewire, but the iliac arteries nearly always resume their former shape without angiographic signs of injury. The rare exceptions are in patients who have rigid arteries that result from severe arterial calcification (Figure 20.2) or retroperitoneal scarring from previous arterial surgery.

One way to make a regular guidewire function as though it were very stiff is to apply traction on both ends, with one end exiting the upper extremity and the other end exiting the lower extremity [3,4]. Unfortunately, traction on the ends of a left brachiofemoral wire is transmitted to the lateral margin of the subclavian orifice, where it can cause arterial rupture. The risk is lessened, but not eliminated, by covering this portion of the wire with a catheter. Alternatively, the right brachial artery can be used for access, but this increases the

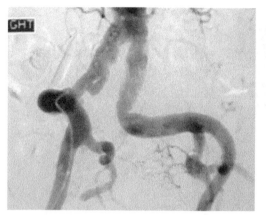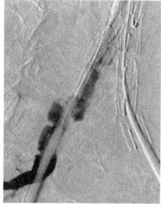

**Figure 20.1** Left, Preoperative angiogram shows tortuosity of the iliac arteries. Right, The stent graft (Zenith AAA endovascular graft; Cook, Inc.) was inserted over a Lunderquist guidewire (Cook, Inc.) without causing permanent arterial injury or distortion.

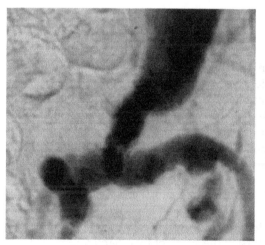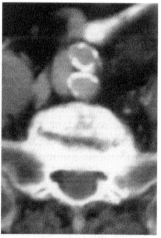

**Figure 20.2** Left, Preoperative angiogram shows iliac tortuosity. Right, Preoperative computed tomographic scan shows associated calcification, which rendered these arteries impassable.

risk of cerebral embolism. In my opinion, ultrastiff wires, such as the Lunderquist guidewire (Cook, Inc., Bloomington, IN), have most of the advantages of a brachiofemoral wire with less risk of bleeding or stroke.

When the arteries are large enough, the entire delivery system can be inserted through a second sheath. The Keller-Timmerman sheath (Cook, Inc.), for example, is more trackable and more kink-resistant than some delivery systems.

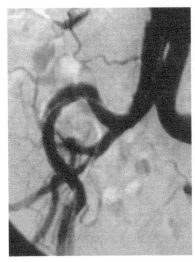 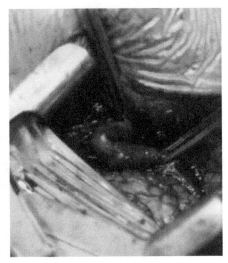

**Figure 20.3** Left, Preoperative angiogram shows tortuosity of the right external iliac artery. Right, Intraoperative photograph shows a redundant loop of external iliac artery that has been pulled down into the groin wound.

The external iliac arteries are usually more tortuous than the common iliac arteries, but they are also easier to straighten. If the inguinal ligament is elevated, digital pressure can be applied to the apex of a loop of the external iliac artery. If this fails, the external iliac artery can be mobilized circumferentially and the redundant loop pulled below the inguinal ligament (Figure 20.3), thereby straightening the segment that remains in the retroperitoneum [5].

A tortuous common iliac artery is more of a problem. Surgical exposure using a retroperitoneal approach is sometimes helpful. The artery may be punctured directly [6] or entered through a prosthetic conduit [7,8]. When a modern delivery system is used, the more important consequences of common iliac tortuosity are its effects on catheter manipulation and graft patency, but these issues are outside the scope of this chapter.

## Aortic tortuosity

Aortic tortuosity is seldom a major impediment to the insertion of a modern delivery system, but older, less trackable systems sometimes stop at the angle between the proximal end of the aneurysm and the distal end of the neck. Under these circumstances, gentle manual pressure is often enough to straighten the aorta and allow the delivery system to pass (Figure 20.4). Potential complications associated with this maneuver, such as arterial disruption and embolism, seem to be rare. If this maneuver fails, one can try bridging the area with a very stiff guidewire or with multiple guidewires from

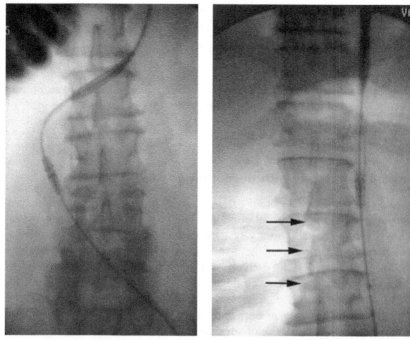

**Figure 20.4** Intraoperative fluoroscopy. Left, Aortic tortuosity is evident by the curved delivery system. Right, Manual pressure applied to the right hypochondrium, in the direction of the arrows, has a straightening effect.

different access sites. Unlike iliac artery tortuosity, aortic tortuosity is not amenable to any direct surgical solution short of conversion to open repair.

## Iliac artery stenosis

Discrete stenosis of the iliac artery may be amenable to angioplasty, with or without a stent. I prefer the Wallstent (Boston Scientific Corp., Natick, MA) because it tends to straighten the artery and it presents a smooth surface to the outer surface of the delivery system. Although heavily calcified orificial lesions maintain the shape of their lumen better with a Palmaz stent (Cordis Corp., Miami, FL), one should remember that the immediate goal is to open a passage for insertion of the delivery system. It is safer and more productive to try to improve the cosmetic results after the stent graft is inserted. Sometimes hydrophilic dilators (Cook, Inc.) and sheaths can be passed through the lesion when the primary delivery systems fail, but this large-scale form of "Dotterization" should be used with caution.

Diffuse stenosis of the external iliac artery is often amenable to endarterectomy through a femoral arteriotomy. A 4F Fogarty balloon occlusion catheter (Edwards Lifesciences Corp., Irvine, CA) provides adequate proximal hemostatic control. Alternatively, one can deliver the stent graft through a surgically created iliofemoral bypass [7,8].

## Aortic stenosis

Distal aortic stenosis and calcification are rarely major obstacles to stent graft insertion. The lesion may complicate insertion of a bifurcated stent graft by compressing the limbs, but the resulting problems and their treatment lie outside the scope of this chapter.

## Surgical compared with percutaneous femoral access

It is always possible to obtain arterial access for endovascular aneurysm repair by percutaneous arterial puncture. The problems occur when one tries to close the hole. Large delivery systems and small, calcified femoral arteries necessitate open surgical repair of the access site. An entirely percutaneous technique is safer when the delivery system is small, the femoral arteries are large and healthy, and a closure device is used to help limit the size of the arterial laceration.

The theoretical advantages of percutaneous repair include the avoidance of anesthesia and the avoidance of surgical wounds. These wounds used to be a major cause of morbidity, but the rate of complications is much lower if one uses small oblique incisions, instead of longitudinal incisions, at the level of the inguinal ligaments [9].

The choice of approach often reflects who is doing the repair. Cardiologists generally prefer percutaneous access because the procedure can be performed in the interventional suite with or without surgical help [10], whereas surgeon-led teams tend to prefer open access because they regard the necessary cutdown as trivial and they feel more comfortable in the operating room.

## Conclusion

Like everything else in endovascular aneurysm repair, the technique of arterial access is device specific. Early-generation devices are not the best choices for anatomically complex iliac arteries; with the use of newer devices, fewer problems are encountered, whatever the pattern of arterial disease. Most importantly, one needs to know the functional limits of the device and select cases accordingly.

## References

1 Moore WS, Vescera CL. Repair of abdominal aortic aneurysm by transfemoral endovascular graft placement. *Ann Surg* 1994; **220**: 331–9.
2 Chuter TA, Reilly LM, Kerlan RK *et al.* Endovascular repair of abdominal aortic aneurysm: getting out of trouble. *Cardiovasc Surg* 1998; **6**: 232–9.

3 Volodos NL, Karpovich IP, Troyan VI *et al.* Clinical experience of the use of self-fixing synthetic prostheses for remote endoprosthetics of the thoracic and the abdominal aorta and iliac arteries through the femoral artery and as intraoperative endoprosthesis for aorta reconstruction. *Vasa Suppl* 1991; **33**: 93–5.

4 Criado FJ, Wilson EP, Abul-Khoudoud O, Barker C, Carpenter J, Fairman R. Brachial artery catheterization to facilitate endovascular grafting of abdominal aortic aneurysm: safety and rationale. *J Vasc Surg* 2000; **32**: 1137–41.

5 Parodi JC. Endovascular repair of aortic aneurysms, arteriovenous fistulas, and false aneurysms. *World J Surg* 1996; **20**: 655–63.

6 Macdonald S, Byrne D, Rogers P, Moss JG, Edwards RD. Common iliac artery access during endovascular thoracic aortic repair facilitated by a transabdominal wall tunnel. *J Endovasc Ther* 2001; **8**: 135–8.

7 Chuter TA, Reilly LM. Surgical reconstruction of the iliac arteries prior to endovascular aortic aneurysm repair. *J Endovasc Surg* 1997; **4**: 307–11.

8 May J, White G, Waugh R, Yu W, Harris J. Treatment of complex abdominal aortic aneurysms by a combination of endoluminal and extraluminal aortofemoral grafts. *J Vasc Surg* 1994; **19**: 924–33.

9 Chuter TA, Reilly LM, Stoney RJ, Messina LM. Femoral artery exposure for endovascular aneurysm repair through oblique incisions. *J Endovasc Surg* 1998; **5**: 259–60.

10 Howell MH, Strickman N, Mortazavi A, Hallman CH, Krajcer Z. Preliminary results of endovascular abdominal aortic aneurysm exclusion with the AneuRx stent-graft. *J Am Coll Cardiol* 2001; **38**: 1040–6.

CHAPTER 21

# Ancillary interventions to provide proximal and distal endograft fixation

**L. Louis Lau, MD, FRCS, Albert G. Hakaim, MD**

## Introduction

Since the first endovascular aneurysm repair (EVAR) in 1991, the number of patients treated with this innovative technique has grown exponentially. After the US Food and Drug Administration approved two devices in 1999, there was a sharp increase in the number of patients with abdominal aortic aneurysm (AAA) being treated with EVAR. It is estimated that >12 000 aortic stent grafts have been implanted worldwide.

Improvements in stent graft design, advanced technical expertise, and increased use of adjunctive intraoperative procedures have all enhanced the applicability and success rate of this minimally invasive approach [1,2]. With various commercial devices and study devices available, up to 60% of patients with AAA can now be treated with EVAR [3,4]. Many of these patients have severe comorbidities and are considered to be at high risk for conventional open repair; others have anatomically complex aneurysms that may render open repair a high-risk procedure. Several published series [2,5,6] suggest that in these patients technical success can be achieved at low risk of morbidity and mortality.

Clearly, EVAR is technically feasible, and the immediate and mid-term results are comparable to those of open aneurysm repair. Immediate conversions to open repair have been rare, and the operative mortality rates are low. The durability and long-term outcome of EVAR remain unclear, however, and long-term follow-up results of prospective randomized trials comparing EVAR and open repair are eagerly awaited. Several studies [7–9] have shown that a clinically significant number of patients initially treated successfully with EVAR required readmission for secondary interventions of procedure-related complications. These complications included early and late endoleaks, graft limb thrombosis, kinking, stent graft migration, and stent fracture. There is also evidence that unplanned adjunctive procedures are being performed intraoperatively during EVAR with increasing frequency [2,10]. This may be the result of improved intraoperative imaging techniques for detecting subtle endoleaks and other problems or of increased technical expertise acquired during the learning curve, which enables physicians to deal with these problems more confidently. Or perhaps it results from a greater awareness that minor intraoperative imperfections may have serious long-term consequences.

Successful endovascular treatment of AAAs requires proximal and distal stent graft fixation to avoid migration and to provide a hemostatic seal, preventing graft-related endoleaks by complete exclusion of the aneurysm from the systemic circulation [11–13]. Technical success is essential to achieving satisfactory immediate and long-term results. The key to technical success in EVAR is preoperative planning with careful selection of the patient and the device. Potential problems can often be anticipated and avoided by screening for anatomical features of the aortoiliac and femoral segments and by paying particular attention to the proximal and distal landing zones. Attention to technical details during the stent graft implantation is paramount, and any intraoperative problems identified should be corrected promptly by using the available resources and endovascular skills. As technical expertise improves, more complex AAAs will be treated by EVAR; therefore, the number of intraoperative technical problems and intraoperative corrections is expected to increase.

Of all the complications encountered in EVAR, proximal or distal type I endoleak is undoubtedly the most worrisome and is the most common type of failure in EVAR [13,14]. Type I endoleak may be detected intraoperatively by arteriography at the time of initial stent graft deployment. Persistent exposure of the aneurysm sac to aortic inflow pressure may lead to continuing aneurysmal expansion, in which case, subsequent rupture is likely. When type I endoleak is detected at the time of the initial operation, there is little disagreement over the need for ancillary interventions to provide a proximal or distal seal and stent graft fixation. The present chapter describes some of the available methods for treatment of type I endoleak, which can be used as intraoperative adjunctive interventions or as secondary procedures.

## Type I endoleak

Type I endoleak indicates a failure of endovascular treatment and represents a persistent risk of aneurysmal rupture. Particularly, proximal type I endoleak is associated with aneurysmal rupture and proximal stent graft migration [13,15]. Analysis from the EUROSTAR (European Collaborators on Stent-Graft Techniques for Abdominal Aortic Aneurysm Repair) database showed that proximal type I endoleak increased the risk of AAA rupture (odds ratio, 10.9; 95% confidence interval, 3.8–30.3) [16]. Various stent grafts were used in the EUROSTAR trial. Nevertheless, it is essential that efforts be directed toward identifying type I endoleak intraoperatively and treating it promptly and effectively by endovascular means. It is generally accepted that no patient should leave the operating room with an unresolved type I endoleak.

The true incidence of intraoperative type I endoleak is difficult to determine because published data are scarce. In a series of 204 patients with AAAs treated with EVAR, 37 patients (18%) developed intraoperative type I endoleak, of which three-quarters were proximal in origin [2]. From the EUROSTAR database of 2146 patients, intraoperative endoleak was observed in 16.7% overall; 3.3% were proximal and 3.6% were distal type I endoleaks. In a smaller study of 33 patients, 30% developed intraoperative proximal endoleak that required adjunctive endovascular interventions [12]. The wide range of the reported incidence may result from different endovascular stent graft devices being used in patients with different anatomical characteristics and from variable performance of completion angiography.

Various anatomical features of the proximal aneurysm neck have been suggested to be risk factors for proximal type I endoleak. The presence of thrombi or calcified atheromatous plaques; a short, conical, or wide neck; and severe neck angulation may be predisposing factors. Albertini *et al.* [15] showed that neck angulation and neck diameter were significantly greater in patients in whom proximal type I endoleak or proximal stent graft migration developed than in patients who had neither of these complications. Multivariate analysis from the EUROSTAR study showed significant correlations between proximal type I endoleak and diameter of the aneurysm neck, proximal aortic neck length, and aortic device diameter [16]. No correlation was identified, however, for neck angulation or for the shape of the aortic neck. In contrast, two retrospective studies did not show any significant association between the aortic neck dimensions and the incidence of proximal type I endoleak [12,17]. When Petrik & Moore [17] retrospectively reviewed their first 100 EVAR patients to identify any preoperative factors that predict endoleak, they were unable to show a statistically significant association with any anatomical characteristics. In a smaller study of 33 patients, Dias *et al.* [12] showed that morphologic features of the aortic neck did not correlate with the incidence of proximal type I endoleak.

Despite these confusing results, physicians at most centers are still cautious and avoid selecting patients with neck morphologic features that are adverse for EVAR, particularly when combinations of those features exist. If the aortic neck length is insufficient to ensure adequate proximal fixation, a suprarenal stent graft may improve the stability but do little to improve the seal. Some authors maintain that this is the most secure form of proximal stent graft fixation [14].

Discrepancies between the type of stent graft and the diameter of the graft vessel at the proximal and distal attachment sites have also been considered important factors for the development of type I endoleak. The EUROSTAR data showed that the rate of proximal type I endoleak decreased as the degree of oversizing increased up to 20%, after which it plateaued. The authors concluded that oversizing the self-expanding stent grafts by at least 10%, and perhaps by even 20%, may help to prevent the occurrence of proximal endoleak [16]. They also found no relationship between different devices and the development of proximal endoleak, although all the devices in the study used self-expanding stents. Generally, oversizing from 10% to 15% is recommended when self-expanding devices are used. This oversizing increases the radial force of the stent graft against the aortic wall, which is vital for fixation. Excessive oversizing may lead to folding of the stent graft fabric and the subsequent appearance of endoleaks [12]. This view is supported by an *in vitro* study showing that oversizing in self-expanding stent grafts resulted in the formation of fabric folds, especially in noncompliant atherosclerotic aortas, and in more serious endoleaks than in balloon-expanded stent grafts. The ability of the self-expanding stent to alter its diameter with each cardiac cycle resulted in a closer relation to the aortic wall during the cardiac cycle, however, and this may accommodate future neck dilation [18]. But if the aortic neck dilates during follow-up, the rigidity of the stent may lead to space developing between the aortic wall and the stent graft, and perigraft endoleak or stent graft migration may result.

Apart from the above-mentioned patient-related and stent graft-related risk factors, technical problems during stent graft deployment may cause proximal type I endoleaks. For example, distal deployment of the stent graft or intraoperative, provoked, downward displacement may occur [15]. In the absence of gross technical error, a type I endoleak represents a failure of patient selection or device selection, or both.

## Management of proximal type I endoleak

When proximal type I endoleak is identified intraoperatively on completion arteriography, the following ancillary endovascular maneuvers, alone or in combination, are useful for improving proximal stent graft fixation: balloon angioplasty, placement of additional stents, placement of extension cuffs, and transcatheter coil embolization (Figure 21.1).

### Balloon angioplasty

If the stent graft is deployed at the proper level, but the seal is inadequate, balloon angioplasty is the most appropriate first step. This maneuver may improve the proximal seal by ensuring full expansion of the device. The mechanism by which balloon angioplasty seals the proximal endoleak of a self-expanding stent graft is not entirely clear. An *in vitro* study showed that balloon angioplasty performed in the presence of fabric folds in the self-expanding stent graft did not affect the amount of folding or the degree of perigraft endoleak [18]. Clinically, devices with hooks and barbs that penetrate the aortic wall may prevent the stent graft from redistributing itself over the aortic surface. The effect of balloon angioplasty may be to realign the graft along the longitudinal axis of the aortic neck rather than to increase the stent graft's radial force, which is limited by the graft fabric. This is particularly true if the aortic neck is angulated and the stent graft separates from the aortic neck. Balloon angioplasty may correct the angulation at the stent attachment site. Fully supported stent grafts offer better columnar strength but at the expense of graft flexibility, which may make them prone to tilting in a tortuous proximal neck, resulting in gaps and perigraft endoleaks. In the presence

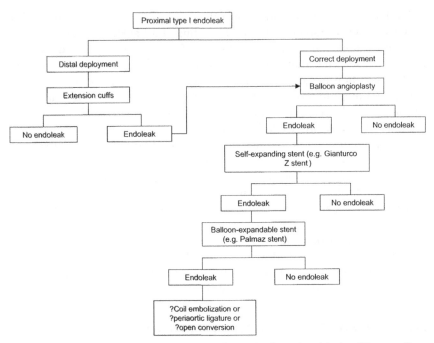

**Figure 21.1** Intraoperative management options for proximal type I endoleaks. (Gianturco Z stent, Cook, Inc.; Palmaz stent, Cordis Corp.)

of a longer neck, balloon angioplasty may allow the stent graft to conform to the neck anatomically and improve the hemostatic seal.

### Additional stents

If balloon angioplasty is not sufficient to achieve a hemostatic seal, application of an additional stent is likely to be successful in resolving the endoleak if the device has been positioned correctly (Figure 21.2). A self-expanding Gianturco Z stent can be deployed within the proximal stent graft or within the bare stent of a transrenal fixation stent graft. This improves the radial force of the stent graft at the proximal fixation site. The self-expanding force of these stents is less than that required for deployment of balloon-expandable stents; however, an advantage of the self-expanding stents is that they do have some elasticity.

The use of a giant Palmaz stent (Cordis Corp., Miami, FL), a balloon-expandable stent, has been reported to improve proximal fixation [12]. The rigidity of the giant Palmaz stents maintains compression on the fabric folds by preventing the recoil of a noncompliant aorta. It also corrects tilting that occurs between the stent graft and a tortuous aortic neck. Theoretically, a potential risk of using this rigid, nonflexible stent is the possibility of acute

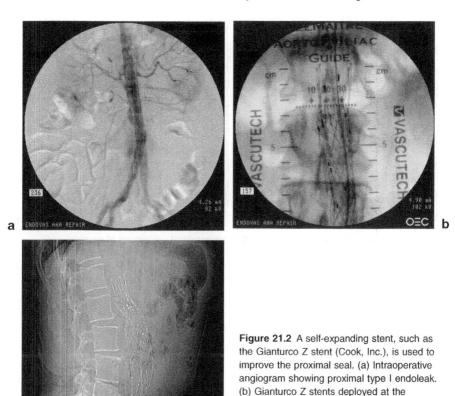

**Figure 21.2** A self-expanding stent, such as the Gianturco Z stent (Cook, Inc.), is used to improve the proximal seal. (a) Intraoperative angiogram showing proximal type I endoleak. (b) Gianturco Z stents deployed at the proximal end of the stent graft. (c) Lateral abdominal radiograph showing the aortic stent graft (AneuRx; Medtronic, Inc.) and Gianturco Z stents.

aortic rupture or damage to the graft fabric. Fortunately, the occurrence of these complications is rare.

## Extension cuffs

When the proximal stent graft is positioned more distally than expected because of misjudgment or migration during deployment, and when there is sufficient length between the renal arteries and the bifurcation of the stent graft, one or more proximal extension cuffs can be placed from the infrarenal aorta to the stent graft to bridge the gap and improve the fixation and hemostatic seal (Figure 21.3). Therefore, during preparation for EVAR, additional devices with various sizes and configurations should be available in the operating room for such use. Extension cuffs are essentially covered stents that are short, so they are relatively expensive to use because additional delivery systems are required. Graft extensions and cuffs can also be used for distal

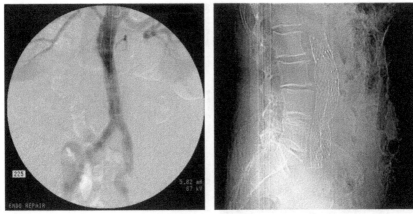

**Figure 21.3** Use of a proximal extension cuff to correct distal deployment of the stent graft.
(a) Angiogram showing distal deployment of the stent graft resulting from misjudgment (note the
distance from the renal arteries to the proximal end of the stent graft). (b) Lateral abdominal
radiograph showing the aortic stent graft and the proximal extension cuff.

perigraft and type IIIa (disjunction of modular stents) endoleaks in a similar
fashion.

## Transcatheter coil embolization

Coil embolization has been used in cases in which there is a well-identified
entry site for the perigraft endoleak and one or more outflow vessels [19]. A
brachial or femoral approach may be used. After embolization of the outflow
vessels, the aneurysm sac is filled with coils in the hope of creating permanent thrombosis. However, in animal studies, coil embolization failed to
decrease intrasac pressure despite resolution of the endoleak, suggesting that
patients may be exposed to a continuing risk of aneurysmal rupture. Therefore, the effectiveness of coil embolization as a treatment of type I proximal
endoleak remains to be proved.

## Open procedures or conversion

Open placement of periaortic ligatures through a transperitoneal incision,
when there is a persistent proximal leak without stent graft migration, has
also been described [2]. This procedure avoids aortic cross-clamping and
may be less invasive hemodynamically than open conversion for high-risk
patients.

Open conversion with proximal and distal aortic clamping is necessary if
the endoleak persists despite the use of the adjunctive endovascular interventions previously mentioned or if the endoleak is associated with proximal
stent graft migration and if adjunctive endovascular techniques are not
feasible. Open conversion is associated with higher mortality rates, especially
in high-risk patients who are not candidates for open repair.

## Management of distal type I endoleak

Poor distal attachment leads to retrograde flow and possibly to distal graft migration proximally into the aneurysm sac. Like proximal endoleak, distal perigraft endoleak poses the same risk of further aneurysmal growth and subsequent rupture, and it should be treated aggressively in a similar manner. Because the distal aorta rarely provides a secure landing zone for distal stent graft fixation, the use of aorto-aortic stent grafts is rarely indicated, except for the repair of juxtarenal anastomotic aneurysm in patients with previous AAA replacement in which the distal landing zone is a graft. Distal type I endoleaks are usually easier to manage with the components of stent grafts. The same general principles apply to the management of distal and proximal type I endoleaks. Balloon angioplasty (Figure 21.4) is usually sufficient if the iliac limb of the stent graft is sized properly and placed in the proper landing zone. If the distal fixation stent has migrated or is malpositioned, extension cuffs or covered stents can be used if the landing zone in the distal common iliac artery is adequate for secure stent graft fixation.

If the above ancillary interventions fail, the hypogastric artery can be sacrificed by coil embolization and the conduit extended into the external iliac artery to ensure an adequate seal. Even though bilateral hypogastric artery occlusion may be tolerated, we prefer to attempt preservation when possible.

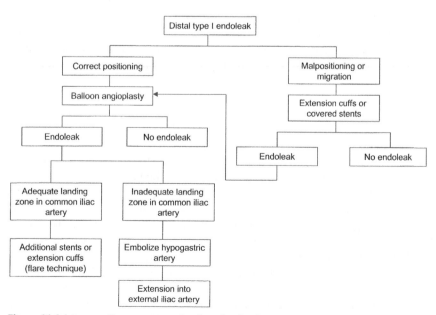

**Figure 21.4** Intraoperative management options for distal type I endoleaks.

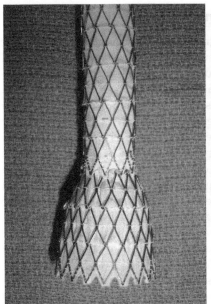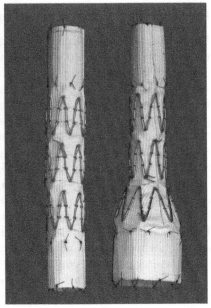

a                                                                                    b

**Figure 21.5** Flared devices. (a) AneuRx aortic extension cuff (Medtronic, Inc.). (b) Flared right
iliac limb of a Zenith bifurcated stent graft (Cook, Inc.).

## The flare technique

Ectatic common iliac arteries are sometimes found in patients with infrarenal
AAA, and most available commercial stent grafts can achieve an adequate
hemostatic seal in iliac arteries that have diameters of no more than 14 mm.
To maintain flow in the hypogastric artery in patients with an ectatic but nonaneurysmal common iliac artery (up to 25 mm in diameter), an AneuRx aortic
extension cuff (Medtronic, Inc., Minneapolis, MN) placed as a distal limb
extension has provided an adequate hemostatic seal in the enlarged vessel
[20,21]. The larger diameter aortic extension cuff is inserted into the distal
portion of the iliac limb of a standard modular bifurcated stent graft, with
flaring of the end of the device into a bell-bottom shape to achieve fixation to
the common iliac artery (Figure 21.5). The diameter of the aortic extension
cuff is oversized by 2–4 mm as compared with the native artery diameter. It
is deployed 1 cm proximal to the origin of the hypogastric artery, preserving
blood flow to the vessel, and with at least 1 cm of overlap with the iliac limb
of the stent graft. The presence of thrombi in the ectatic common iliac artery
suggests aneurysmal change and is considered a contraindication for this
technique. The long-term durability of this technique is uncertain because it
is not known whether subsequent enlargement of the ectatic common iliac
arteries occurs.

At Mayo Clinic, Jacksonville, Florida, between November 1999 and November 2000, we used this distal flare technique in 15 patients (19 vessels) who

had ectatic common iliac arteries (diameter range, 15–25 mm) and were undergoing EVAR using bifurcated modular devices. We used two types of commercially available stent graft devices with distal flared cuffs (distal flare diameter, 18–28 mm), AneuRx and Zenith (Cook, Inc.) (Figure 21.5). All AAAs were successfully excluded with no open conversion or perioperative mortality. At 12-month follow-up with contrast-enhanced computed tomography, all AAAs remained excluded, with no evidence of distal type I endoleak or graft migration. There was no significant change in the diameter of the common iliac arteries at 6 months, and follow-up is continuing to assess the long-term durability of this technique [22].

If the common iliac artery is aneurysmal or lined with thrombi, a stent graft extension is required in the normal external iliac artery after coil embolization of the hypogastric artery. The technique is not without complications, and disabling buttock claudication, colonic ischemia, and sexual dysfunction have been described.

## Conclusions

Endovascular stent graft repair of AAA is an exciting, evolving field in vascular surgery. As physicians gain experience and stent graft designs improve, more high-risk patients with complex aneurysms are being treated with this minimally invasive technique. Intraoperative problems are becoming more frequent and additional endovascular interventions are often required. Therefore, physicians involved in the treatment should be proficient in advanced endovascular skills so that they can use adjunctive procedures efficiently whenever intraoperative problems arise.

## References

1  Resch T, Malina M, Lindblad B, Ivancev K. The evolution of Z stent-based stent-grafts for endovascular aneurysm repair: a life-table analysis of 7.5-year followup. *J Am Coll Surg* 2002; **194**(Suppl): S74–8.

2  Kalliafas S, Albertini JN, Macierewiecz J *et al*. Incidence and treatment of intraoperative technical problems during endovascular repair of complex abdominal aortic aneurysms. *J Vasc Surg* 2000; **31**: 1185–92.

3  Carpenter JP, Baum RA, Barker CF *et al*. Impact of exclusion criteria on patient selection for endovascular abdominal aortic aneurysm repair. *J Vasc Surg* 2001; **34**: 1050–4.

4  Woodburn KR, Chant H, Davies JN, Blanshard KS, Travis SJ. Suitability for endovascular aneurysm repair in an unselected population. *Br J Surg* 2001; **88**: 77–81.

5  Chuter TA, Reilly LM, Faruqi RM *et al*. Endovascular aneurysm repair in high-risk patients. *J Vasc Surg* 2000; **31**: 122–33.

6  Buth J, van Marrewijk CJ, Harris PL, Hop WC, Riambau V, Laheij RJ, for the EUROSTAR Collaborators. Outcome of endovascular abdominal aortic aneurysm repair in patients with conditions considered unfit for an open procedure: a report on the EUROSTAR experience. *J Vasc Surg* 2002; **35**: 211–21.

7  Carpenter JP, Baum RA, Barker CF *et al*. Durability of benefits of endovascular versus conventional abdominal aortic aneurysm repair. *J Vasc Surg* 2002; **35**: 222–8.

8 Makaroun MS, Chaikof E, Naslund T, Matsumura JS. Efficacy of a bifurcated endograft versus open repair of abdominal aortic aneurysms: a reappraisal. *J Vasc Surg* 2002; **35**: 203–10.

9 Sternbergh WC III, Carter G, York JW, Yoselevitz M, Money SR. Aortic neck angulation predicts adverse outcome with endovascular abdominal aortic aneurysm repair. *J Vasc Surg* 2002; **35**: 482–6.

10 Resch T, Malina M, Lindblad B, Ivancev K. The impact of stent-graft development on outcome of AAA repair: a 7-year experience. *Eur J Vasc Endovasc Surg* 2001; **22**: 57–61.

11 White GH, Yu W, May J, Chaufour X, Stephen MS. Endoleak as a complication of endo-luminal grafting of abdominal aortic aneurysms: classification, incidence, diagnosis, and management. *J Endovasc Surg* 1997; **4**: 152–68.

12 Dias NV, Resch T, Malina M, Lindblad B, Ivancev K. Intraoperative proximal endoleaks during AAA stent-graft repair: evaluation of risk factors and treatment with Palmaz stents. *J Endovasc Ther* 2001; **8**: 268–73.

13 Chuter TA, Faruqi RM, Sawhney R *et al.* Endoleak after endovascular repair of abdominal aortic aneurysm. *J Vasc Surg* 2001; **34**: 98–105.

14 Chuter TA. Stent-graft design: the good, the bad and the ugly. *Cardiovasc Surg* 2002; **10**: 7–13.

15 Albertini J, Kalliafas S, Travis S *et al.* Anatomical risk factors for proximal perigraft endoleak and graft migration following endovascular repair of abdominal aortic aneurysms. *Eur J Vasc Endovasc Surg* 2000; **19**: 308–12.

16 Mohan IV, Laheij RJ, Harris PL, for the EUROSTAR Collaborators. Risk factors for endoleak and the evidence for stent-graft oversizing in patients undergoing endovascular aneurysm repair. *Eur J Vasc Endovasc Surg* 2001; **21**: 344–9.

17 Petrik PV, Moore WS. Endoleaks following endovascular repair of abdominal aortic aneurysm: the predictive value of preoperative anatomic factors: a review of 100 cases. *J Vasc Surg* 2001; **33**: 739–44.

18 Schurink GW, Aarts NJ, van Baalen JM, Schultze Kool LJ, van Bockel JH. Stent attach-ment site-related endoleakage after stent graft treatment: an in vitro study of the effects of graft size, stent type, and atherosclerotic wall changes. *J Vasc Surg* 1999; **30**: 658–67.

19 Golzarian J, Struyven J, Abada HT *et al.* Endovascular aortic stent-grafts: transcatheter embolization of persistent perigraft leaks. *Radiology* 1997; **202**: 731–4.

20 Brown DB, Sanchez LA, Hovsepian DM, Rubin BG, Sicard GA, Picus D. Use of aortic cuffs to exclude iliac artery aneurysms during AneuRx stent-graft placement: initial expe-rience. *J Vasc Interv Radiol* 2001; **12**: 1383–7.

21 Karch LA, Hodgson KJ, Mattos MA, Bohannon WT, Ramsey DE, McLafferty RB. Man-agement of ectatic, nonaneurysmal iliac arteries during endoluminal aortic aneurysm repair. *J Vasc Surg* 2001; **33**(Suppl): S33–8.

22 Hakaim AG, Lau LL, Neuhauser B *et al.* A comparison of AneuRx aortic cuff and Zenith distal flare exclusion of common iliac artery ectasia for endovascular aneurysm repair. *Vasc Endovasc Surg* 2004; **38**: 51–6.

# CHAPTER 22

# Prevention, diagnosis, and management of endoleaks

Srinivasa Rao Vallabhaneni, MD, FRCS, Martin Malina, MD, PhD, Björn Sonesson, MD, PhD, Krassi Ivancev, MD, PhD

## Introduction

Endovascular repair attempts to prevent rupture of an aneurysm by isolating the aneurysm from both blood flow and blood pressure. Despite endovascular repair, in some patients blood continues to flow within the aneurysm. This phenomenon of blood flow within the aneurysm but outside the stent graft is termed endoleak [1,2]. Initially, because the significance of endoleak was uncertain, there were various opinions and practices related to its management. Over the years, however, several aspects of endoleak have been investigated in both clinical and laboratory studies, so that now the immediate and long-term consequences of endoleak are better understood.

Endoleaks are classified according to the origin of blood flow (Table 22.1) [3]. It is also usual to further qualify each type of endoleak to provide more information, such as primary (present since the endovascular repair), secondary (appearing later, after the endovascular repair), or delayed (discovered after prior negative imaging); transient or persistent; and treated. This chapter aims to provide an overview of prevention, diagnosis, and management of different types of endoleak according to the prevailing consensus and evidence.

## Clinical significance

The clinical significance of endoleak is best examined in relation to the role it might play in negating the primary purpose of endovascular repair, namely, prevention of aneurysmal rupture. Functionally an endoleak has two components, the blood flow within the endoleak and the pressure an endoleak might transmit to the aneurysm sac. The main consideration is that pressure on the aneurysm sac alone can cause rupture. The consequences of rupture, however, depend on the rate of blood flow within the endoleak channel because the rest of the circulation has been isolated from the aneurysm. Perfusion within an aneurysm does not necessarily mean that the aneurysm sac

**Table 22.1** Classification of endoleaks.

| Endoleak type | Source of blood flow |
| --- | --- |
| I* | Attachment site |
| a | Proximal end of stent graft |
| b | Distal end of stent graft |
| c | Iliac occluder |
| II | Branch vessel |
| a | Simple or to-and-fro (from 1 patent branch) |
| b | Complex or flow-through (2 or more patent branches) |
| III* | Stent graft defect |
| a | Modular junctional leak |
| b | Fabric disruption (i.e., hole) |
| | Minor (<2 mm; e.g., suture hole) |
| | Major (≥2 mm) |
| IV | Stent graft fabric porosity |

*Types I and III are generally referred to as graft-related endoleaks.
(Modified and reprinted from Veith FJ, Baum RA, Ohki T *et al.*, Nature and significance of endoleaks and endotension: summary of opinions expressed at an international conference. *J Vasc Surg* 2002; **35**: 1029–35, Copyright 2002, with permission from The Society for Vascular Surgery.)

is exposed to systemic pressure. Conversely and more importantly, significant pressurization of the aneurysm sac may occur in the absence of a demonstrable endoleak.

## Detection

Endoleak can be detected by various imaging methods. Gadolinium-enhanced magnetic resonance angiography and microbubble-enhanced duplex ultrasonography can be used effectively to identify endoleaks during surveillance [4,5]. Although both methods avoid exposure to ionizing radiation and nephrotoxic contrast material, the former is limited by incompatibility with certain stent graft models and the latter is disadvantaged by its operator dependency. The purpose of postoperative surveillance imaging, however, includes gathering information about several other aspects of the state of aneurysm repair in addition to the detection of endoleak. Computed tomography (CT) is the best compromise for this purpose and is the mainstay of postoperative surveillance. Triple-phase contrast-enhanced CT is widely used as the benchmark to judge the sensitivity and specificity of other methods of endoleak detection [6]. Angiography with selective catheterization, however, is required in selected patients to rule out low-flow endoleak or to define an endoleak track accurately.

It is not always possible to be certain that an endoleak does not exist owing to limitations of the diagnostic methods. It is also occasionally difficult to image an endoleak in sufficient detail for accurate classification. More than one type of endoleak may coexist. Although such coexistence is often obvious when present, it may mislead. For example, a patent aortic side branch functioning as an outflow channel for a graft-related endoleak may appear to be a simple type II endoleak on standard surveillance imaging.

## Graft-related endoleaks (type I and type III)

The consequences of type I and type III endoleaks are identical: they result in exposure of the aneurysm directly to systemic blood pressure and to potentially high rates of blood flow, creating a high risk of aneurysmal rupture. These are detected on routine surveillance (dual-phase CT). The patient is also likely to present with symptoms or rupture owing to sudden pressurization of the aneurysm sac. There is evidence that the majority of late ruptures after endovascular repair are associated with a graft-related endoleak [7]. An aneurysm sac that has been excluded may lose its strength, and sudden repressurization from a delayed graft-related endoleak can precipitate rupture. It is also known that graft-related endoleaks are harbingers of serious outcome unless treated, even if they have disappeared spontaneously after an apparently benign course [8–10]. The prevailing consensus is that graft-related endoleaks should be remedied immediately [3].

## Primary type I endoleak

A primary endoleak from an attachment site occurs when there is poor apposition between the native blood vessel and the fabric of the stent graft at the sealing zones. This occurs when an aneurysm is anatomically adverse or a stent graft is used incorrectly; the reported incidence varies widely. Anatomical factors reported to be significantly associated with a higher risk of a primary type Ia endoleak include short aneurysm neck (<10 mm), severe angulation of the neck (>50°), large diameter of the neck (>30 mm), and the presence of calcification within the neck [11,12]. The risk of a proximal type I endoleak is also increased when the neck contains atheromatous plaque or ridges and when the neck is conical and has large aneurysms. Maldeployment of a stent graft so as not to overlap the entire length of available neck, reducing the effective neck length, also increases the risk of an endoleak [12]. Standard practice is to use a stent graft with a diameter that is 10–20% larger than the aneurysm neck diameter (oversizing). Too much oversizing can result in fabric folds that create channels for endoleak, but placing a stent graft that is too small for the native vessel will not provide a seal. All these factors hamper effective and adequate contact between the stent graft fabric and the native vessel. Distal attachment site endoleaks also occur for similar reasons. Appropriate selection of patients and devices, together with accurate deployment, is therefore the key to prevention of type I endoleak.

Diagnosis of a primary type I endoleak is made on completion angiography. Both detection and definition of subtle endoleaks are enhanced by good-

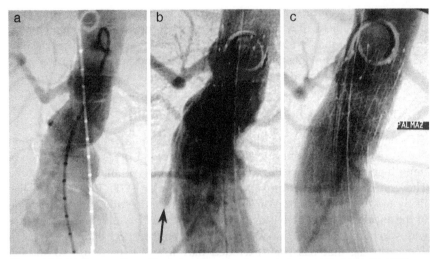

**Figure 22.1** (a) Preoperative calibrated angiography demonstrated a conical and angulated aneurysm neck. (b) Completion angiography revealed a proximal type I endoleak (arrow). (c) The endoleak was successfully remedied by the placement of a large-diameter Palmaz stent (Cordis Corp.).

quality equipment. All components of the angiographic protocol, such as catheter positions, contrast medium injections, views from multiple angles, frame rate of image acquisition, and total duration of each sequence, significantly influence the quality of angiography but are often underestimated. Analysis of the intrasac pressure wave by means of an indwelling catheter can aid detection of a graft-related endoleak [13,14]. Absence of a graft-related endoleak is usually associated with a decrease in the intrasac pulse pressure. Persistence of a pulse pressure greater than half of the systemic pulse pressure is indicative of a graft-related endoleak. This method appears to be sensitive and specific but is not widely used for clinical purposes.

The general consensus is that no patient should leave the operating table with a primary proximal type I endoleak (type Ia) [3]. Distal type I endoleaks (type Ib) are perceived to be less dangerous, but it is good practice to remedy these also at the time of the primary endovascular repair. If the stent graft has been positioned correctly, treatment of a primary proximal type I endoleak involves balloon dilatation of the anastomotic zones, and often that is all that is necessary. If this fails, a balloon-expandable stent (e.g., a Palmaz stent; Cordis Corp., Miami, FL) can be used to improve both alignment and contact between the stent graft and the native vessel and to obliterate any channels within fabric folds. Large Palmaz stents are highly effective in correcting such endoleaks but carry a small risk of causing arterial rupture (Figure 22.1). When the stent graft has been maldeployed, a proximal type I endoleak can be treated by using an extension cuff.

## Secondary and delayed type I endoleak

The exact incidence of secondary and delayed type I endoleak remains unknown but seems to be low with newer generation stent grafts. Proximal fixation and seal are maintained by the stent graft's radial force and columnar strength. Postoperative aneurysm neck dilatation [15] and structural disintegration of the stent graft [16] can compromise these factors, predisposing to stent graft migration and endoleak. Fixation appendages incorporated at the proximal stent graft, such as hooks or barbs, enhance and preserve fixation significantly [17].

Dilatation or aneurysmal change of the iliac vessel landing zones and hemodynamic displacement forces result in the loss of distal fixation and cephalad migration of the iliac limbs [18,19]. Newer stent grafts are designed to minimize this risk. The entire length of the common iliac artery should be used as a landing zone to reduce the risk of endoleak, and stent graft limbs should be extended into the external iliac artery when a common iliac artery is aneurysmal. If it is necessary to extend stent grafts into the external iliac arteries on both sides, the use of a branched stent graft to preserve perfusion of at least one internal iliac artery is preferable to covering both internal iliac arteries. Covering both internal iliac arteries results in gluteal claudication and, rarely, skin or bowel necrosis.

Since a delayed type I endoleak is usually precipitated by stent graft migration, all surveillance images should be assessed routinely and methodically to detect any migration of the proximal stent graft. Minor degrees of migration may suggest loss of fixation and may herald a more serious and precipitous migration. Migration occurring by small increments may be overlooked when comparisons are made between surveillance images from the last two intervals only. To avoid this, the latest images should always be compared with the earliest images. Because the course of migration is unpredictable, any degree of migration should prompt a thorough evaluation of the situation. The possible need for a prophylactic secondary intervention should be considered even when a seal is preserved by the remaining overlap between the stent graft and the landing zone.

When associated with migration, treatment of a type Ia endoleak involves placing an extension cuff. In selected patients, a fenestrated extension can be deployed to extend the seal zone proximally while preserving the visceral blood flow. This technique is complex, requiring a custom-made device, and stent graft models with shorter bodies may not have enough space to accommodate a fenestrated cuff. When not associated with migration, a large-diameter Palmaz stent may be used. Closing type I endoleak tracks by injecting thrombosing agents or placing coils has been abandoned because of concerns with pressure transmission through a thrombus. When endovascular intervention is not possible, application of a periaortic ligature by open surgery has also been reported, a technique that is not always successful. Distal type I endoleaks are usually easier to manage, and endovascular insertion of a limb extension is almost always successful. Removal of the stent graft and conversion to open repair of the aneurysm is the definitive option when other methods are not feasible or successful. Conversion to open repair is associated with considerable mortality, and it should be the last resort.

## Type III endoleak

An endoleak occurring from discontinuity between the modular components of a stent graft or from a defect in the fabric is a rare but serious condition. A primary type III endoleak may result from maldeployment of a modular component. Modular disconnection during follow-up may result from morphologic changes in the aneurysm and stent graft distortion. A distorted (kinked) stent graft limb is also exposed to increasing hemodynamic distractional forces that aid modular disconnection. Newer-generation modular devices have an enhanced strength of fixation between components, and manufacturers' guidance for the minimal acceptable overlap between components must always be followed during the operation. Erosion of fabric owing to constant cyclical friction between the fabric and the stent struts may result in fabric holes. This is expedited in the presence of sharp ends of fractured stents [16]. Several modifications have been incorporated into stent graft design lately, including the use of thicker fabric and suture-free methods of binding the stent struts to the fabric, leading to a reduction in the incidence of this complication. Correction of a type III endoleak involves placing a stent graft to bridge the modular components or to cover the fabric defect as necessary.

## Type IV endoleak

The interstices within the stent graft fabric may allow contrast material to flow across the fabric soon after deployment, resulting in type IV endoleak. Its incidence depends on the type of stent graft. Type IV endoleak is detected on completion angiography or on early CT that may have been done for various reasons. This type of endoleak resolves spontaneously with deposition of fibrin and platelets soon after implantation. Type IV endoleak should not be diagnosed beyond 30 days after stent graft placement [3].

## Type II endoleak

### Type II endoleak on completion angiogram

Primary type II endoleak is common. The main consideration is its distinction from a graft-related endoleak. The possibility that a type II endoleak is a marker of a hidden graft-related endoleak should always be considered. The importance of intraoperative imaging in this regard has already been alluded to. Type II endoleaks always appear late in the angiographic sequence because of the retrograde nature of the blood flow. Primary type II endoleaks do not require intervention because a high proportion of them resolve spontaneously with no adverse effect.

## Type II endoleak during follow-up

There is growing evidence that the incidence of type II endoleaks in late follow-up is dependent on the make and model of the stent graft, although the exact mechanism by which this occurs has not been elucidated [20]. In theory, preoperative obliteration of all infrarenal aortic side branches should result in virtual freedom from type II endoleak. When this has been attempted, though, technical difficulties have made it impossible to embolize all side branches in all patients [21]. Filling the aneurysm sac with thrombogenic sponge at the time of endovascular repair was reported to be effective in preventing type II endoleak, but this procedure did not gain widespread acceptance [22].

There is evidence that the probability of type II endoleak is higher when there are more patent side branches preoperatively. Therefore, preoperative embolization of the inferior mesenteric artery and accessory renal arteries has been advocated when they are associated with multiple patent lumbar arteries [23]. Large side branches with a potential for high retrograde flow, such as the internal iliac artery (when the stent graft sealing zones are within the external iliac artery), should be preoperatively embolized to reduce the risk of a type II endoleak. Coils are used most frequently for embolization; particulate material is avoided owing to the risk of distal ischemia.

The influence of type II endoleaks on the long-term efficacy of endovascular repair varies among patients, and uncertainties exist in several areas, leading to differences in approaches to management. Isolated type II endoleak has been incriminated rarely as the sole cause of a late rupture [24]. More frequently, type II endoleak is associated with expansion or absence of shrinkage of the aneurysm during follow-up. Expansion of the aneurysm creates a risk of continued anatomical distortion, leading to loss of fixation and graft-related endoleak with consequent danger. Therefore, type II endoleak should be treated in an expanding aneurysm. Any other possible coexisting causes of aneurysmal enlargement should be investigated and ruled out.

Aneurysms may shrink in the presence of type II endoleaks [25]. It is reasonable in such circumstances to continue using a conservative approach. The problem of a persistent type II endoleak when the size of the aneurysm remains the same is a subject of controversy. A pragmatic approach that allows tailored management appropriate for individual patients is one that takes into consideration factors such as the size of the aneurysm, the state of the seal zones, the feasibility of a successful secondary intervention, and the patient's general health. Selection of patients for secondary intervention based on direct measurement of intrasac pressure through translumbar puncture has also been reported.

Treatment of type II endoleak involves occlusion of the blood vessels forming the flow circuit. Reducing the number of vessels in the circuit is often adequate to disrupt the endoleak without targeting all the vessels. Infrarenal aortic side branches may be selectively catheterized for coil embolization. It is possible to reach the main trunk of an inferior mesenteric artery using

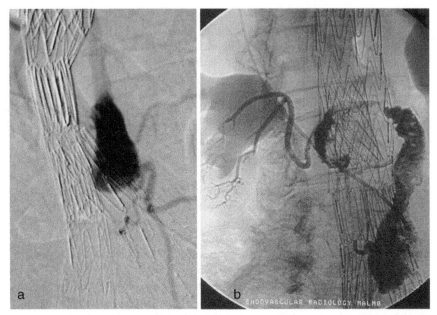

**Figure 22.2** (a) Translumbar puncture of the enlarging aneurysm revealed a persistent type II endoleak. (b) Contrast angiography demonstrated the full extent of the endoleak circuit, which included an unsuspected communication between an accessory renal artery and lumbar arteries. The endoleak was successfully treated with glue injection.

coaxial microcatheters through the superior mesenteric artery or through the ileolumbar collaterals. Direct puncture of the aneurysm through a percutaneous translumbar approach to access the endoleak channel and embolization with different agents have been reported [26,27] (Figure 22.2). An important complication of this intervention is inadvertent embolization of arteries and distal ischemia.

A conventional surgical approach to the side branches and ligation is also an established intervention. A transperitoneal laparoscopic approach to ligate a patent inferior mesenteric artery and various other conventional surgical approaches that aim to preserve the stent graft have been described to abolish troublesome type II endoleaks [28,29].

## Expansion of aneurysm free from endoleak

The aneurysm may expand despite apparent freedom from endoleak. Sometimes this results from limitations of the imaging methods; selective and exhaustive angiography may reveal a low-flow endoleak in some patients. Intermittent endoleaks that evade detection have also been proposed as an explanation. It is well established that transmission of pressure can occur without actual blood flow and that recurrent or persistent pressurization of the aneurysm sac (endotension) can lead to enlargement or even rupture of the aneurysm [30,31]. Several potential routes of pressure transmission other than endoleak have been identified. Laminated thrombi and atheromas can transmit pressure, and areas of native vessels lined with them should not be used as landing zones. Pressure can also be transmitted through microleaks in the body of the graft or in the graft material and through thrombosed endoleaks. The term "hygroma of the aneurysm sac" has been used to describe aneurysms that are free from endoleak and that appear to enlarge from the accumulation of fluid at relatively low pressures [32].

Management options in these circumstances are often limited and unclear because of ambiguity regarding the source of pressurization or cause of enlargement and difficulties in accurately estimating the risk of rupture in individual patients with the conservative approach. Conversion to open repair should be considered in all these patients to avoid rupture.

## Conversion to open repair

The majority of endoleaks can be treated successfully with endovascular techniques, and some ruptures associated with graft-related endoleak can also be treated with endovascular methods. Conversion to open repair is required in situations such as failed treatment of graft-related endoleak, failed treatment of type II endoleak in the presence of aneurysmal expansion, and expansion of an aneurysm free from endoleak.

## References

1 White GH, Yu W, May J, Chaufour X, Stephen MS. Endoleak as a complication of end-luminal grafting of abdominal aortic aneurysms: classification, incidence, diagnosis, and management. *J Endovasc Surg* 1997; **4**: 152–68.
2 White GH, May J, Waugh RC, Chaufour X, Yu W. Type III and type IV endoleak: toward a complete definition of blood flow in the sac after endoluminal AAA repair. *J Endovasc Surg* 1998; **5**: 306–9.
3 Veith FJ, Baum RA, Ohki T *et al*. Nature and significance of endoleaks and endotension: summary of opinions expressed at an international conference. *J Vasc Surg* 2002; **35**: 1029–35.
4 Haulon S, Lions C, McFadden EP *et al*. Prospective evaluation of magnetic resonance imaging after endovascular treatment of infrarenal aortic aneurysms. *Eur J Vasc Endovasc Surg* 2001; **22**: 62–9.
5 McWilliams RG, Martin J, White D *et al*. Detection of endoleak with enhanced ultrasound imaging: comparison with biphasic computed tomography. *J Endovasc Ther* 2002; **9**: 170–9.
6 Fillinger MF. New imaging techniques in endovascular surgery. *Surg Clin North Am* 1999; **79**: 451–75.
7 Fransen GA, Vallabhaneni SR Sr, van Marrewijk CJ, Laheij RJ, Harris PL, Buth J, EUROSTAR. Rupture of infra-renal aortic aneurysms after endovascular repair: a series from EUROSTAR registry. *Eur J Vasc Endovasc Surg* 2003; **26**: 487–93.
8 Mialhe C, Amicabile C, Becquemin JP, Stentor Retrospective Study Group. Endovascular treatment of infrarenal abdominal aneurysms by the Stentor system: preliminary results of 79 cases. *J Vasc Surg* 1997; **26**: 199–209.

9 Skillern CS, Stevens SL, Piercy KT, Donnell RL, Freeman MB, Goldman MH. Endotension in an experimental aneurysm model. *J Vasc Surg* 2002; **36**: 814–7.
10 Mehta M, Ohki T, Veith FJ, Lipsitz EC. All sealed endoleaks are not the same: a treatment strategy based on an ex-vivo analysis. *Eur J Vasc Endovasc Surg* 2001; **21**: 541–4.
11 Mohan IV, Laheij RJ, Harris PL, EUROSTAR Collaborators. Risk factors for endoleak and the evidence for stent-graft oversizing in patients undergoing endovascular aneurysm repair. *Eur J Vasc Endovasc Surg* 2001; **21**: 344–9.
12 Sampaio SM, Panneton JM, Mozes GI *et al.* Proximal type I endoleak after endovascular abdominal aortic aneurysm repair: predictive factors. *Ann Vasc Surg* 2004; **18**: 621–8.
13 Vallabhaneni SR, Gilling-Smith GL, How TV *et al.* Aortic side branch perfusion alone does not account for high intra-sac pressure after endovascular repair (EVAR) in the absence of graft-related endoleak. *Eur J Vasc Endovasc Surg* 2003; **25**: 354–9.
14 Chaudhuri A, Ansdell LE, Grass AJ, Adiseshiah M. Intrasac pressure waveforms after endovascular aneurysm repair (EVAR) are a reliable marker of type I endoleaks, but not type II or combined types: an experimental study. *Eur J Vasc Endovasc Surg* 2004; **28**: 373–8.
15 Dillavou ED, Muluk S, Makaroun MS. Is neck dilatation after endovascular aneurysm repair graft dependent? Results of 4 US phase II trials. *Vasc Endovasc Surg* 2005; **39**: 47–54.
16 Guidoin R, Marois Y, Douville Y *et al.* First-generation aortic endografts: analysis of explanted Stentor devices from the EUROSTAR Registry. *J Endovasc Ther* 2000; **7**: 105–22.
17 Resch T, Malina M, Lindblad B, Malina J, Brunkwall J, Ivancev K. The impact of stent design on proximal stent-graft fixation in the abdominal aorta: an experimental study. *Eur J Vasc Endovasc Surg* 2000; **20**: 190–5.
18 Mohan IV, Harris PL, Van Marrewijk CJ, Laheij RJ, How TV. Factors and forces influencing stent-graft migration after endovascular aortic aneurysm repair. *J Endovasc Ther* 2002; **9**: 748–55.
19 Liffman K, Lawrence-Brown MM, Semmens JB, Bui A, Rudman M, Hartley DE. Analytical modeling and numerical simulation of forces in an endoluminal graft. *J Endovasc Ther* 2001; **8**: 358–71.
20 Ouriel K, Clair DG, Greenberg RK *et al.* Endovascular repair of abdominal aortic aneurysms: device-specific outcome. *J Vasc Surg* 2003; **37**: 991–8.
21 Gould DA, McWilliams R, Edwards RD *et al.* Aortic side branch embolization before endovascular aneurysm repair: incidence of type II endoleak. *J Vasc Interv Radiol* 2004; **12**: 337–41.
22 Walker SR, Macierewicz J, Hopkinson BR. Endovascular AAA repair: prevention of side branch endoleaks with thrombogenic sponge. *J Endovasc Surg* 1999; **6**: 350–3.
23 Axelrod DJ, Lookstein RA, Guller J *et al.* Inferior mesenteric artery embolization before endovascular aneurysm repair: technique and initial results. *J Vasc Interv Radiol* 2004; **15**: 1263–7.
24 Hinchliffe RJ, Singh-Ranger R, Davidson IR, Hopkinson BR. Rupture of an abdominal aortic aneurysm secondary to type II endoleak. *Eur J Vasc Endovasc Surg* 2001; **22**: 563–5.
25 Gilling-Smith GL, Martin J, Sudhindran S *et al.* Freedom from endoleak after endovascular aneurysm repair does not equal treatment success. *Eur J Vasc Endovasc Surg* 2000; **19**: 421–5.
26 Rial R, Serrano FJ, Vega M *et al.* Treatment of type II endoleaks after endovascular repair of abdominal aortic aneurysms: translumbar puncture and injection of thrombin into the aneurysm sac. *Eur J Vasc Endovasc Surg* 2004; **27**: 333–5.

27 Baum RA, Carpenter JP, Golden MA *et al.* Treatment of type 2 endoleaks after endovascular repair of abdominal aortic aneurysms: comparison of transarterial and translumbar techniques. *J Vasc Surg* 2002; **35**: 23–9. Erratum in: *J Vasc Surg* 2002; **35**: 852.

28 Ho P, Law WL, Tung PH, Poon JT, Ting AC, Cheng SW. Laparoscopic transperitoneal clipping of the inferior mesenteric artery for the management of type II endoleak after endovascular repair of an aneurysm. *Surg Endosc* 2004; **18**: 870.

29 Lipsitz EC, Ohki T, Veith FJ *et al.* Delayed open conversion following endovascular aortoiliac aneurysm repair: partial (or complete) endograft preservation as a useful adjunct. *J Vasc Surg* 2003; **38**: 1191–8.

30 Gilling-Smith G, Brennan J, Harris P, Bakran A, Gould D, McWilliams R. Endotension after endovascular aneurysm repair: definition, classification, and strategies for surveillance and intervention. *J Endovasc Surg* 1999; **6**: 305–7.

31 White GH, May J, Petrasek P, Waugh R, Stephen M, Harris J. Endotension: an explanation for continued AAA growth after successful endoluminal repair. *J Endovasc Surg* 1999; **6**: 308–15.

32 Risberg B, Delle M, Lonn L, Syk I. Management of aneurysm sac hygroma. *J Endovasc Ther* 2004; **11**: 191–5.

# PART V

## Appendix

# Reporting standards for endovascular aneurysm repair

## Albert G. Hakaim, MD

The results of any surgical technique must be compared among surgeons and medical centers. Given the relatively new technique of endovascular aneurysm repair (EVAR), and the consequent development of complications and situations unique to it, a system of uniform reporting standards is essential. Regardless of the background of the practitioner or the venue of device deployment, placement of a graft for EVAR must be viewed as the beginning of a lifelong commitment between the patient and the physician. As emphasized throughout this monograph, the majority of postoperative complications with EVAR are usually asymptomatic at detection and are only discovered with vigilant, scheduled patient imaging and physical examination. In addition, endoleaks may first appear or reappear years after EVAR. The purpose of this appendix is to briefly review the published standards of clinical specialists who perform EVAR and provide postoperative follow-up.

In 1997, the need for reporting standards after EVAR was initially addressed. These early attempts at standardization were largely patterned after the standards applied to traditional vascular surgical procedures. The main focus was primary and secondary patency and classification of the cause of the aneurysm. Also reported at that time were the first attempts to characterize persistent flow into the excluded aneurysm segment, or endoleak. Initially, endoleaks were classified as primary (demonstrated on completion angiogram or first computed tomographic scan); secondary (not detected early); or recurrent (after an endoleak had been sealed) [1]. Also at that time, the Society for Vascular Surgery and the International Society for Cardiovascular Surgery published their recommendations for risk stratification based on aortoiliac anatomy [2].

As experience with EVAR and follow-up imaging increased, further refinements in endoleak classification followed. Specifically, the classification expanded from type I and type II endoleaks to include type III (fabric defect, inadequate modular seal, or modular disconnection) and type IV (graft porosity causing "a blush"). In addition, endopressure, or nonendoleak aneurysm sac pressurization, was first described. Unlike an endoleak of unknown cause, "endopressure" referred to a situation in which the aneurysm sac exhibited systemic pressure or continued to increase in diameter without a demonstrable endoleak [3].

With increased acceptance of EVAR as a viable option for infrarenal aneurysm repair, reporting standards were refined further. A second report was published from the Ad Hoc Committee for Standardized Reporting Practices in Vascular Surgery of the Society for Vascular Surgery/American Association for Vascular Surgery [4]. This publication provides a detailed description of the accepted standards for reporting all aspects of endovascular aneurysm repair, including the following excerpt:

> *Initial* or *30-day clinical success* encompasses 30-day data. *Short-term clinical success* includes outcome measures reported within a 30-day to 6-month time frame. *Mid-term clinical success* refers to all outcome measures that are statistically significant up to 5 years after endograft implantation. *Long-term clinical success* includes all outcome measures that are statistically significant beyond 5 years.

It is again emphasized that, following EVAR, surveillance imaging and clinical visits must continue throughout the patient's life.

Further refinement in the definition and classification of endoleaks has been an ongoing process. In 2002, a summary of world opinion regarding the nature and significance of endoleaks and endotension was published [5]. A refined classification scheme for endoleaks and endotension was described and is illustrated in Table A-1. The utility of this detailed classification is evidenced by its repeated citation in the literature [6,7]. Of interest, the original description of endopressure has now been redefined as endotension with four subtypes. Recently, endotension has been implicated in >5% of patients after EVAR [6].

As has been detailed elsewhere in this monograph, the cornerstone of imaging before and after EVAR is the computed tomographic (CT) scan. As CT imaging has become further refined, its application has undergone evolution as well. Initially, thin-cut, conventional dynamic CT scanning was the primary technique used. Spiral CT scanning has, however, become the preferred technique [8]. Although it is essential that patients receive follow-up imaging, this has led to concern about repetitive exposure to ionizing radiation and potentially nephrotoxic iodinated intravenous contrast media. The frequency of such imaging is variable, depending on the practitioner. A schedule of 1-month, 6-month, and then biannual studies seems to be prudent for patients in whom an endoleak has not been detected or treated. If the aneurysm sac has been completely reabsorbed, or if the size of the aneurysm has been stable for 24 months, consideration is given to annual CT scanning or biannual duplex imaging to assess maximal aneurysm sac diameter. As an alternative to the potentially detrimental effects of CT scanning, magnetic resonance imaging with gadolinium enhancement has been shown to be at least as sensitive as spiral CT scanning for the detection of type II endoleaks [6].

Recent experimental efforts have focused on measurement of intrasac pressure before and after EVAR. In a bench model, intrasac pressure was repro-

**Table A-1** Classification of endoleaks and endotension.

| Type of endoleak | Source of perigraft flow |
| --- | --- |
| I | Attachment site |
| a | Proximal end of graft |
| b | Distal end of graft |
| c | Iliac occluder |
| II | Branch leaks |
| a | 1 patent branch |
| b | 2 or more patent branches |
| III | Graft defect |
| a | Junctional leak or modular disconnection |
| b | Fabric disruption |
|  | Minor (<2 mm; e.g., suture hole) |
|  | Major (≥2 mm) |
| IV | Graft porosity |
| Endotension |  |
| a | With no endoleak |
| b | Following sealing of endoleak |
| c | With type I or III endoleak* |
| d | With type II endoleak* |

*Detectable only on opening the aneurysm sac.
(Modified and reprinted from Veith FJ, Baum RA, Ohki T *et al.*, Nature and significance of endoleaks and endotension: summary of opinions expressed at an international conference. *J Vasc Surg* 2002; **35**: 1029–35, Copyright 2002, with permission from The Society for Vascular Surgery.)

ducibly reduced following stent graft placement. With the creation of a type I endoleak, these pressures increased significantly. The introduction of a type II endoleak did not, however, significantly change intrasac pressure waveforms [8]. The application of transcutaneous sac pressure monitoring may play a role in the detection of type I endoleaks.

Early clinical experience with pulsatile wall motion measurement has recently been reported. These measurements were made using an electronic echo-tracking device, interfaced with a B-mode real-time ultrasound scanner, and a linear array transducer. A series of 162 patients treated over a 9-year period were analyzed. Pulsatile wall motion was permanently decreased in all patients after successful aneurysm exclusion. At present, pulsatile wall motion measurement lacks the sensitivity to detect all endoleaks [9].

## References

1 Rutherford RB. Reporting standards for endovascular surgery: should existing standards be modified for newer procedures? *Semin Vasc Surg* 1997; **10**: 197–205.
2 Ahn SS, Rutherford RB, Johnston KW *et al.*, Ad Hoc Committee for Standardized Reporting Practices in Vascular Surgery of the Society for Vascular Surgery/International Society

for Cardiovascular Surgery. Reporting standards for infrarenal endovascular abdominal aortic aneurysm repair. *J Vasc Surg* 1997; **25**: 405–10.

3 White GH, May J, Waugh RC, Chaufour X, Yu W. Type III and type IV endoleak: toward a complete definition of blood flow in the sac after endoluminal AAA repair. *J Endovasc Surg* 1998; **5**: 305–9.

4 Chaikof EL, Blankensteijn JD, Harris PL *et al.*, Ad Hoc Committee for Standardized Reporting Practices in Vascular Surgery of the Society for Vascular Surgery/American Association for Vascular Surgery. Reporting standards for endovascular aortic aneurysm repair. *J Vasc Surg* 2002; **35**: 1048–60.

5 Veith FJ, Baum RA, Ohki T *et al.* Nature and significance of endoleaks and endotension: summary of opinions expressed at an international conference. *J Vasc Surg* 2002; **35**: 1029–35.

6 Choke E, Thompson M. Endoleak after endovascular aneurysm repair: current concepts. *J Cardiovasc Surg (Torino)* 2004; **45**: 349–66.

7 Pearce WH. What's new in vascular surgery. *J Am Coll Surg* 2003; **196**: 253–66.

8 Geller SC, Society of Interventional Radiology Device Forum. Imaging guidelines for abdominal aortic aneurysm repair with endovascular stent grafts. *J Vasc Interv Radiol* 2003; **14**: S263–4.

9 Chaudhuri A, Ansdell LE, Grass AJ, Adiseshiah M. Intrasac pressure waveforms after endovascular aneurysm repair (EVAR) are a reliable marker of type I endoleaks, but not type II or combined types: an experimental study. *Eur J Vasc Endovasc Surg* 2004; **28**: 373–8.

# Index

Note: page numbers in *italics* refer to figures, those in **bold** refer to tables.

Printed and bound by CPI Group (UK) Ltd, Croydon, CR0 4YY

16/04/2025

14658822-0003